WOMBS IN LABOR

SOUTH ASIA ACROSS THE DISCIPLINES

SOUTH ASIA ACROSS THE DISCIPLINES

EDITED BY MUZAFFAR ALAM, ROBERT GOLDMAN,
AND GAURI VISWANATHAN

DIPESH CHAKRABARTY, SHELDON POLLOCK,
AND SANJAY SUBRAHMANYAM, FOUNDING EDITORS

Funded by a grant from the Andrew W. Mellon Foundation and jointly published by the University of California Press, the University of Chicago Press, and Columbia University Press

South Asia Across the Disciplines is a series devoted to publishing first books across a wide range of South Asian studies, including art, history, philology or textual studies, philosophy, religion, and the interpretive social sciences. Series authors all share the goal of opening up new archives and suggesting new methods and approaches, while demonstrating that South Asian scholarship can be at once deep in expertise and broad in appeal.

For a list of books in the series, see page 253.

WOMBS IN LABOR

TRANSNATIONAL COMMERCIAL SURROGACY IN INDIA

 AMRITA PANDE

COLUMBIA UNIVERSITY PRESS   NEW YORK

Columbia University Press

Publishers Since 1893

New York   Chichester, West Sussex

cup.columbia.edu

Library of Congress Cataloging-in-Publication Data

Pande, Amrita.

Wombs in labor : transnational commercial surrogacy in India / Amrita Pande.

pages cm. — (South Asia across the disciplines)

Includes bibliographical references and index.

ISBN 978-0-231-16990-5 (cloth : alk. paper) —

ISBN 978-0-231-16991-2 (pbk. : alk. paper) —

ISBN 978-0-231-53818-3 (e-book)

1. Surrogate motherhood—India.   2. Surrogate mothers—India.   I. Title.

HQ759.5.P36 2014

306.874'3—dc23

2014004973

Columbia University Press books are printed on permanent
and durable acid-free paper.

This book is printed on paper with recycled content.

Printed in the United States of America

c 10 9 8 7 6 5 4 3 2 1

p 10 9 8 7 6 5 4 3 2 1

Cover photograph: Miriam Hinman Nielsen

Cover design: Lisa Hamm

To Didu, my maternal grandmother

CONTENTS

ACKNOWLEDGMENTS

THIS BOOK could not have been possible without the nurturance of many people. Foremost are the women who consented to be interviewed and shared their tears, laughter, and surrogacy stories with me. Most of these women must remain anonymous. But no less important are those who can and must be named. My academic advisors, angels, knights in shining armor: Millie Thayer, Robert Zussman, Joya Misra, and Elizabeth Hartmann in Amherst, Massachusetts, not only gave help with the contents of this book but also fortified my spirit with their emotional support through all the crises that inevitably inundate a writer's life. Their support and advice, concerning not just the book but anything else that might have affected my sanity, have kept pouring in despite the physical distance between us. I cannot thank you enough. I am indebted to Michael Burawoy and Arlie Hochschild for their unexpected and insightful feedback on early drafts of some chapters. This project would have been impossible to complete without two generous fellowships provided by the Social Science Research Council and one by the University of Massachusetts, Amherst, as well as a research development grant by the University of Cape Town, South Africa.

Fellow panelists at several conferences and editors and reviewers of journals pushed me along with key questions on some of this material. A number of articles based on this project have been published in journals. Part of chapter 4 appeared in 2010 in *Signs: Journal of Women in Culture and Society* 35 (4): 969–94. Part of chapter 5 appeared in 2011 in *Reproductive BioMedicine Online* 23 (5): 618–25. Part of chapter 7 appeared in 2010 in *Feminist Studies*, Special Issue on Reproduction and Mothering, 36 (2): 292–312, and in 2009 in *Indian Journal of Gender Studies* 16 (2): 141–73.

Finally, part of chapter 8 was published in 2009 in *Qualitative Sociology* 32 (4): 379–405. I am grateful to the fellow panelists, the journal editors, and anonymous and known reviewers for all their feedback—the good, the bad, and the ugly.

As they say in Bollywood movies, friendship means "No thank you, no sorry!" So, study buddies, fellow sufferers, and my surrogate family in Amherst, Massachusetts—Annette Hunt, Anne Hector, Brittnie Aiello, Emmanuel (Manny) Adero, Jiye Kim, Kat Jones, Kathleen Hulton, Martha Morgan, Sofia Checa, and Swati Birla—here are all the accumulated "Thank yous" and "Sorrys" that I never said. My enthusiastic group of critics and friends in Tripoli, Lebanon, deserve more than a mention. Oliver Bridge, Joana Cameira, Sara Dominoni, Nancy Hilal, and Elsa Salame asked the right questions at the right time, and encouraged me to make this manuscript a "readable read." My current home, Cape Town, offered a fresh batch of critics, colleagues, and friends. Amna Khalid, Elena Moore and the Sitas-Von Kotze family (Ari Sitas, Astrid Von Kotze, Rike Sitas) brainstormed with me about many versions of new chapters. Their impromptu suggestions over cups of coffee and bottles of wine helped me and the book stay afloat during my first few years at the University of Cape Town. Other colleagues and friends at UCT—David Lincoln, David Cooper, John De Gruchy, Lucy Earle, and Nancy Odendaal—gave occasional feedback on these new chapters. I am grateful to the SSRC-Mellon Book Fellowship for keeping the book on track and introducing me to Adi Hovav, the most patient editor-reader of the first few drafts of this book. Series editor Gauri Viswanathan and Jennifer Crewe, my editor at Columbia University Press, impressed me with their frank advice throughout the process. Again, many thanks for keeping the faith. A special thanks to Jan McInroy for her wonderful copyediting skills and for gently persuading me to use "persuade" instead of "convince"!

This book and research got a fresh lease on life in 2009 when I started interacting with Ditte Marie Bjerg, the creative head of Global Stories, a Danish theater company that works on projects lying at the intersection of gender and globalization. Our experiments with interactive theater have taken us all around the globe, and finally back to the surrogates in India. Thanks, Ditte, for embarking on this adventure with me!

Heartfelt thanks to Akhil and Manisha Kumar for their affection and heroic patience. Their kind query "Have you reached the conclusion yet?" served as one of the best deadlines. Ishita played a crucial role not only as the persuasive elder sister who coaxed a weary economist to become a sociologist instead but also as a mentor and successful book author. Our daily writing sessions over brownies and cups of coffee at the Harvard Coop in Cambridge and at Café Lazari in Cape Town helped me meet many deadlines, cheerfully.

There are never enough words to thank one's parents. So I won't even try thanking my parents, Bratati and Shailendra Pande, for their boundless affection, unfaltering support, and determined praise for everything I do.

Something much more than thanks is due to my partner in crime, Aditya Kumar, for indulging me with the kind of love, wisdom, and patience that only he is capable of. It is true; I couldn't have done this without you. Zaira, you enter the stage as I add the final touches to this book. I was told your arrival would change the whole meaning of this project for me. As I sneakily type these lines between the hourly feeds and after the sleepless nights, I have to confess that it did indeed.

WOMBS IN LABOR

1 ❧ INTRODUCTION

WOMBS IN LABOR

The instruments of this labor, or the bodily means of production, . . . are the hands and the head, but never the womb or the breasts of a woman.

—Maria Mies, *Patriarchy and Accumulation on a World Scale*

I N FEBRUARY 2006 I came across a short newspaper article in the *Guardian* about the emergence of a new industry in India (Ramesh 2006). Surrogacy, the article stated, was "India's new form of outsourcing," where couples from all over the world could hire Indian women to bear their children for a fraction of the cost of surrogacy elsewhere and with no government regulations. I confess that the news article unsettled me. Flashes of Margaret Atwood's fictional city in *The Handmaid's Tale* passed through my mind, where a class of women is valued merely as breeders of children of the privileged race and class. Perhaps India was where Atwood's fears would come true, where skinny Indian women would be kept captive in dormitories like the handmaids-in-training, where they would sleep on old military cots and would be watched continuously by matrons with cattle prods.[1] As a fresh immigrant to the United States, constantly battling against orientalized images of India, I found myself haunted even more by these chilling visions. Was my country gradually becoming a land of not just slum dogs, call centers, and yogis but also baby farms? After some digging around, I soon realized that there was scarcely any comprehensive research about this new form of outsourcing, and so began my ethnographic journey into the first country in the global south to have a flourishing industry in both national and transnational surrogacy.

Field notes, 2006, Armaan Maternity Clinic, Garv, India:[2] The room is lined with eight beds, one next to the other with barely enough space to walk in between. A ceiling fan groans above. Some of the beds are raised on one side with a block so that the women can have their legs elevated after the embryo transfer or any gynecological checkups. There is nothing else in the room. Each bed has a pregnant woman resting on it. This is their home for the next few months. Their husbands can visit, but not stay the night. It's a reminder that they cannot have sex. Not for the next few months. The women are still in their nightclothes, and it's nearly evening. The day has been planned for them, the morning visit from the doctor, 8 am breakfast, 9 am medicines, 10 am rest hour, 12 pm injections, followed by an afternoon nap. The evening is nothing different. Except perhaps the broker will bring in a new member. A bed will be added to the room. Another pregnant woman will join the ranks.

Field notes, 2007, Armaan Maternity Clinic, Garv, India: It feels strange to be back. Last year when I went to say goodbye, the doctor asked me rather bluntly, "You are not going to be back, right?" I said, "No" and meant it. But here I am, back in the clinic. . . . The doctor is surprisingly welcoming and waves out a "Hi" through her pink sleeveless T-shirt. Last year she was always wrapped in a traditional Indian *sari* and this new avatar is intriguing. I wonder if it has anything to do with her starring in Oprah Winfrey's segment on infertility. On the doctor's instructions, a nurse leads me to the new wing of the clinic—a brand-new surrogacy hostel. It is their rest hour but the surrogates agree to talk if I sneak in some snacks for them. I run down and get *dhokla-chaat* [baked dough with raisins] and we gather around the first bed to devour the food. I feel disturbed that the surrogates are still given such little space and absolutely no privacy in this new hostel. But as I watch their camaraderie I wonder, "Are they perhaps better off lying next to each other, chatting and laughing their bizarre pregnancy away?"

Field notes, 2011, Surrogacy Hostel, Garv, India: Here I am, five years after the journey had begun. I expect things to be different. After all, surrogacy has now spread from this clinic in Garv to almost any metropolis in India you can name. There is yet another twist in the tale—I am revisiting the field in my sixth month of pregnancy. The surrogate mothers have decided to organize a *godh bharai* [a Hindu ceremony similar to a baby shower] for me. In some parts of India a *godh bharai* ceremony is ritually performed for pregnant women in their seventh month of pregnancy. The hostel matron organizes such a ceremony for all surrogates irrespective of their religion, and the intended parents pay for it. For my ceremony, Durga takes full charge of getting me dressed up like an Indian bride. She gets my costume ready—an ornate pink sari, perfect for the occasion. Jaya is nominated as the "priest" as she is the only upper-caste woman around. The women pray and sing songs to Lord Ganesh (God of Prosperity) and Matarani (Mother goddess). As the singing continues, a surrogate Vaishali quietly remarks, "The only difference is that at the end of it all you get to keep the baby."

SURROGACY TALES

Commercial surrogacy is a topic not restricted to medical circles. It has been generating feminist, ethical, legal, and social debates for more than three decades. This scholarship can be loosely classified into four frames: liberal feminist defense of the practice that emphasizes a woman's right to use her body as she chooses (Andrews 1988; Andrews and Douglass 1991), works that debate the ethics or morality of this practice (Anderson 1990; Bailey 2011; Brennan and Noggle 1997; Oliver 1989; Radin 1987), feminist literature that focuses on the multiple systems of stratification that are potentially reinforced by such practices (Corea 1986; Dworkin 1978; Harding 1991; Neuhaus 1988; Raymond 1993; Roberts 1997; Rothman 1988), and more recent ethnographic scholarship on the impact of surrogacy on the meanings of motherhood, kinship, and work (Franklin and Roberts 2006; Hochschild 2012; Markens 2007; Pande 2009a, 2009b, 2010; Rudrappa 2012; Teman 2010; Vora 2012). Although the recent "ethnographic turn" in the scholarship has diluted the "moral certainty" about the need to reject surrogacy practices, the overwhelming response continues to be one of intense anxiety (Bailey 2011).[3]

The anxiety surrounding commercial surrogacy increases multifold when surrogacy involves women in the global south. Until recently, the predominant focus of much of the debate on surrogacy centered on the practice in the global north, especially in Europe and North America. This is not altogether surprising, since commercial surrogacy is a very recent phenomenon in the global south. The complete absence of any empirical data, however, did not prevent scholars from making alarming predictions about "wombs sans frontiers," especially when the wombs belonged to women in the global south (Sengupta 2010, 8). For instance, Andrea Dworkin predicted in 1978: "While sexual prostitutes sell vagina, rectum and mouth, reproductive prostitutes would sell other body parts: wombs, ovaries and eggs" (quoted in Corea 1986, 275), and Barbara Katz Rothman asked in 1988: "Can we look forward to baby farms, with white embryos grown in young and Third world women?" (100).[4] Indeed, on the long flight from Boston to India, with Gena Corea's *The Mother Machine* (1986) on artificial insemination and artificial wombs as my sole companion, baby farms seemed like compelling metaphors for surrogacy in India.

But over the course of the five years during which I sat by the bedsides of the surrogates listening to their stories, praying with them, and cooking lunches for them in the surrogacy hostel, I came to realize that my textbook and Eurocentric understanding of commercial surrogacy was going to be entirely inadequate for this new and unusual setting for surrogacy in India. At first glance surrogacy in India may well resemble what philosopher Alison Bailey (2011) labels a "feminist dystopian novel," but sustained interactions with the women involved, from the doctor who ran the clinic to the intended mothers and the surrogates themselves, would unravel my assumptions about the nature of surrogacy. This would give way to a more nuanced understanding of the impact of new reproductive technologies on women of the global south as well as a more complex theorization of the intersections of reproduction, labor, and globalization.

In 2006 when I discussed my research project with friends and colleagues, most recoiled with horror at what globalization and new technologies have made possible. Many wondered why they had not heard about this stunning new form of outsourcing, where poor women who are often from the global south are renting their wombs to people from the global north. Since 2010, this phenomenon has started generating some thought-provoking academic discussion (Bailey 2011; DasGupta and Das DasGupta 2010; Hochschild 2012; Rudrappa 2012; Twine 2011; Vora 2012).[5] In fact, every week I receive at least one query from a graduate student, researcher, or scholar across the world who is interested in interviewing surrogates in India. The popular media (both in India and outside) have not been left behind. Pick up the right issue of the *Wall Street Journal*, *Mother Jones*, the *New York Times*, *Marie Claire*, or even better, switch to the right television channel, and you will get an update on surrogacy in India. An Oprah Winfrey segment on surrogacy clinics in India spread the news so effectively that it increased some clinics' international clientele exponentially. Invariably these media reports on surrogacy start with a description of the crowded streets, the filth, and the pigs going through trash outside the clinic, and then move on to the swollen stomachs of

these enterprising-although-illiterate Indian women and to their life stories filled with drunken husbands and desperate poverty. The reporters
note the not insignificant cost difference of surrogacy in India and in the
United States (surrogacy in India costs about a third of what it costs in
the United States). The Indian women in these journalistic accounts are
almost uniformly portrayed as grateful recipients of the opportunity to
serve as surrogates and earn more money than they would earn in more
than ten years. The cameras give us a close-up of a shy smile on the face
of the surrogate, a wider smile on the doctor's face, and a final shot of
the beaming California mother holding her chubby newborn. It seems to
be a happy ending for them all. Of course, today's video images are more
convincing than the predictions made by radical feminists a few decades
ago. But what happens when the cameras stop rolling?

It would be a mistake to attribute commercial surrogate mothering
to a simple synergy of needs of two classes of women—one group the
affluent in India or abroad, needing healthy wombs, and the other group,
needing money. This formulation fails to account for the actors outside
of the client-surrogate mother-baby triad and ignores the dynamics of
surrogacy outside the sphere of reproduction. Indeed, the surrogate
mother negotiates a novel kind of relationship with the baby and the
intended mother. But commercial surrogates in India are navigating
much more than their identity as mothers. They are grappling with their
new identity as participants in a fledgling market in India that is morally
contentious and constructed as deviant and unnatural in mainstream
Indian society. While some of these women are coerced into surrogacy
by their families, many others are negotiating with their families to
gain control over their own bodies and their fertility in order to participate in this process. As surrogates, they suddenly find themselves in an
unfamiliar relationship with a hyper-medicalized system of reproduction, a medical system that has previously been inaccessible to them as
lower-class women in an anti-natalist state. This hyper-medicalization of
reproduction within surrogacy inevitably implies that these women are
simultaneously grappling with the surveillance of their bodies and other
disciplining tactics used by the clinic. Finally, as women hired by clients
from within and across borders, they are straddling complex relationships that often cross boundaries of race, class, and nationality. A linear
emphasis on the reproduction and mothering component of commercial
surrogacy discounts these intricacies of surrogacy in the Indian context.
Instead of burying surrogacy within the usual debates of motherhood and

reproduction, *Wombs in Labor* analyzes commercial surrogacy as a form of labor that traverses the socially constructed dichotomy between production and reproduction. I demonstrate that commercial surrogacy in India is a new kind of labor emerging with globalization: gendered, exceptionally corporeal, and highly stigmatized, but labor nonetheless.

WAGES FOR WOMBS

Feminist scholars have previously used the analogy of "labor" and/or "production" for surrogacy, very often to condemn the commodification of women and motherhood in the process of this labor. Anthropologist Emily Martin discusses medical metaphors whereby the uterus becomes a machine and the woman becomes the laborer that produces the baby. Technology and patriarchy, according to Martin, together produce a "depersonalized mother machine being manipulated to efficiently produce babies out of valued sperm" (quoted in Rothman 2000, 34). Legal scholar Kelly Oliver uses the term "estranged labor" to argue that "surrogacy is the quintessence of capitalist patriarchy's estranged construction of motherhood" (1989, 112). Surrogates, unlike other women who sell their bodies, perform their bodily service nonstop and are, in essence, "never off-duty" (1989, 98). Barbara Katz Rothman, in a similar critique of how technology and patriarchy intersect to oppress women, has argued that "as babies and children become products, mothers become producers, pregnant women the unskilled workers on a reproductive assembly line" (2000, 6). Rothman seems to be critical of the use of the language of work for mothering. She believes that this reduces the intimate and emotional experience. As motherhood becomes work, and children the product of the labor of mothering, Rothman argues, there is "commodification of children and the proletarianization of motherhood" (39). In a more recent study, Jyotsna Agnihotri Gupta (2012, 27) introduces an interesting twist to the analogy of labor when she labels surrogacy as the "industrialization of motherhood" and surrogates as "co-producers" (and not just consumers, as with contraceptives). Curiously, Gupta quickly abandons this language of "co-production" by women and resorts to an often used analogy of organ trade and human trafficking: "While trafficking in solid organs, and sex tourism involving women and children and human trafficking, is considered morally reprehensible, abhorrent, and is penalized, trade in reproductive body parts and exploiting women as surrogates have become socially acceptable practices" (47).

The commodification of women's reproductive labor or what sociologist Eileen Boris and Rhacel Salazar Parreñas (2010) call *intimate* labors—whether domestic work, sex work, care work or, in the case of surrogacy, "womb work"—produces such intense anxieties as it allows for the extension of the market into the private and intimate sphere of sexuality and reproduction.[6] Surrogacy, in particular, is troubling to many because it defies laws of nature, family, and religion, and is perceived to be a commercialization of children, motherhood, and the act of giving birth. The assumption underlying such anxieties is that while human labor may be bought and sold, women's reproductive labor is intrinsically not a commodity (Anderson 1990; Satz 1992; Warnock 1985). The bond between a mother and her child is assumed to be fundamentally different from the bond between a worker and his or her product, and the commercialization of these intimate ties is believed to be degrading for both the mother and the baby.[7] Carole Pateman (1988) suggests a slightly modified version of this argument by claiming that a woman's reproductive labor is "more integral" to her identity than her other productive capacities and hence should be treated differently (207). Elizabeth Anderson (1990) adds that the commodification of reproductive labor makes pregnancy an alienated form of labor for the women who perform it: selling her reproductive labor alienates a woman from her "normal" emotions.

Central to these claims are some fundamental assumptions about children, mothers, and reproductive labor—the uncontested "pricelessness" of children, the "natural" biological bases of reproductive labor, and the related assumption that women's reproduction belongs to a sacred, special realm. The priceless child, however, is a historical construction. Paid parenting and the alleged commodification of children are not new to societies. In the classic book *Pricing the Priceless Child*, Viviana A. Zelizer (1985) writes about instances of paid parenting in the United States in the nineteenth and early twentieth centuries—boarding mothers (foster mothers who agreed to take care of a child in state-subsidized homes), baby farmers (who were paid by parents to look after their illegitimate children), and wet nurses. Zelizer traces how, over time, laws in the United States removed children from the marketplace. Much like the priceless child is a historical construction, the mother-child bond is a social rather than a "natural" creation. As philosopher Debra Satz (2010, 122) succinctly puts it: "Not all women bond with their fetuses. Some women abort them." Nor do all mothers bond with their children naturally. Maternal bonding and affection are culturally and socially determined, and a mother-child relationship often evolves over time.

While it's not surprising that markets in reproductive labor are more troubling than other labor markets, I am disturbed by the implicit reification of gender-based dichotomies—private/public, nature/social, reproduction/production, and non-market/market—in many arguments against surrogacy. These rigid and gendered distinctions have been long identified as the basis of the asymmetrical and patriarchal division of labor where the concept of labor is reserved for men's productive work while women's share in production and reproduction becomes a function of their biology and nature. Ironically, in such a conceptualization, the act of giving birth, or "labor," is implicitly assumed to be not labor or work but rather an activity of nature. In her pioneering work on the sexual division of labor, Maria Mies (1986) contends that to challenge the asymmetrical division of labor it is critical that women's activity in bearing and rearing children be understood as a conscious social activity—that it be understood as work. By conceiving of commercial surrogacy (giving birth for pay) as "labor," *Wombs in Labor* challenges these gendered dichotomies by analyzing the social and historical context under which these dichotomies are undone. I choose the word "labor" over "work" because the word "labor" is used to describe both work (especially hard physical work) often undertaken as a means of earning income and the process of childbirth. These two definitions overlap in the case of commercial surrogacy, where labor becomes the capacity to produce and reproduce in order to earn a living.

Commercial surrogacy evokes such intense moral anxieties that debates find it hard to veer from the morality of the practice. But in India, where surrogacy is fast emerging as a survival strategy and a temporary occupation for some poor rural women, it makes little analytical sense to *simply* battle about morals in abstraction. To paraphrase critical theorist Nancy Fraser, a feminist critique that is "merely a defensive project and that seeks to protect women's reproductive labor from the sphere of market" is both inadequate and inappropriate (SAMA 2012, 29).[8] By conceptualizing commercial surrogacy as labor it is possible to arrive at a much more accurate and nuanced analysis. Such a frame moves beyond the moral sensibilities of the researcher and beyond the moral perception of the unnaturalness of a labor market in wombs to a more analytical question— a question about how a labor market for wombs is created and how the laborers experience this market. By identifying commercial surrogacy as labor, susceptible like other kinds of labor to exploitation, and simultaneously recognizing the women as laborers, *Wombs in Labor* complicates the image of the victim that is inevitably evoked whenever bodies of Third World women are in focus. In her provocative book *Varat och varan* (Being and the Commodity), Swedish author and social commentator Kajsa Ekis Ekman (2011) compares surrogacy to prostitution and gives a caustic critique of what she believes is the neoliberal imperative to "ban the victim" in both of these industries. This abolition of the victim is allegedly a step toward legitimizing inequalities between classes and sexes. In making the claim that commercial surrogacy in India is a new form of labor, and that the surrogates are laborers and not mere victims, I do not ignore the multiple bases of inequality in this form of labor. It cannot be denied that the limited range of a surrogate's alternative economic opportunities and the unequal power relations between the client and the surrogate call into question the voluntary nature of this labor. But instead of dismissing the labor market as inherently oppressive and the women involved as subjects of this oppressive structure, there is need to recognize, validate, and systematically evaluate the choices that women make in order to participate in that market. A comprehensive evaluation of these choices, in turn, reveals the many intersecting layers of domination impinging on them.[9]

Finally, this frame allows for comparisons between surrogacy in India and other forms of women's labor—a comparison of the character of these markets and the forms in which compliance with a labor regime is enforced and resisted, at the level of the family, the clinic, and the state. Commercial surrogacy is a remarkable instance of reproductive labor, where production and reproduction not only intersect but collapse into each other. This extreme intersection shapes the labor regime—the recruitment and disciplinary tactics used by the medical staff—but also the surrogates' strategies for negotiating and resisting this regime.

WOMBS, WORK, AND EVERYDAY RESISTANCE

The study of resistance should not focus on the bow (an ostensible act of obeisance to power) nor the fart (a covert act of resistance to power) but rather on the ways in which these intersect in the moment to produce complex and often contradictory dynamics of control and resistance.

—Dennis K. Mumby, "Theorizing Resistance in Organization Studies"

Since the 1970s, anthropologists, sociologists, political scientists, and feminists alike have been bravely confronting the monolithic formulation of the hegemonic process as something that excludes alternatives to the current structure of power. Whether the floodgates were opened by E. P. Thompson's (1978) study of eighteenth-century English society or James Scott's (1985) analysis of everyday resistance by Malay peasants is debatable. But across disciplines, scholars have been preoccupied with recovering even the most unlikely forms of subversions by the oppressed: small and local resistances, often remaining at the discursive level and not tied to the overthrow of systems or even to ideologies of emancipation (Abu-Lughod 1990, 42).[10] Indeed, identifying subversive acts has become so much in vogue that everything from spectacular revolutions to gossiping has been described as resistance. Despite the contribution of this scholarship to the widening of our definition of the political, it has not escaped criticism. It seems that in our enthusiasm to recover resistances we have inadvertently drawn too strict a contrast between the oppressive world of power and the liberating world of resistance—what Lila Abu-Lughod aptly terms the "romance of resistance" (42). Matters, however, are much more complex and ambivalent. Power and resistance are connected in multiple, complex, and unexpected ways, and resistance often either mimics or reinscribes alternative forms of power.

During the course of my research into the surrogacy market in India, I observed unexpected and sometimes exhilarating instances of everyday resistances by the surrogates to the regime that aimed to control and discipline them. Although it is tempting to merely highlight the ability of this group of women to resist, subvert, and challenge, my primary intention is to demonstrate how the surrogates' resistance to one set of forces inevitably involves reification of other forms of domination. The women's resistances to the multiple layers of domination—by the state, the clinic, and their families—draw attention to the twin paradoxes of the study. The first paradox speaks to India's history of anti-natalism and low rates of medicalization of reproduction. How does a labor market based on pronatal technologies fit in the context of an aggressively anti-natalist state? How do we analyze the sudden hyper-medicalization of childbirth for a class of women who typically have little or no access to the medical system? *Wombs in Labor* demonstrates that as surrogates negotiate with power at the micro level of the family and the clinic, their resistive strategies inadvertently speak to these contradictions at the macro level of the state and its politics. The second paradox highlighted by the many instances of everyday resistances speaks to the "labor" frame of analyzing surrogacy in India. Despite my determined focus on surrogacy as labor, the real laborers in this study, the surrogates themselves, either actively or inadvertently resist classifying surrogacy as labor and themselves as laborers. Each chapter reveals powerful instances of discursive strategies used by the surrogates to subvert the disciplinary regime of the clinic, challenge the stigmatizing labels by the community and media, or question control by the family. Surrogates equate surrogacy to the "divine," reassert control over their "productive bodies," construct moral boundaries between themselves and prostitutes and baby-sellers, and forge kinship ties with the fetus, intended mothers, or other surrogates. But seldom do they speak of surrogacy as a labor option, or construct themselves as laborers. In fact, the protagonists, reproduce the very dichotomies that I, as a researcher, challenge in this book. Their discursive strategies ultimately reify the predominant role of women as virtuous reproducers rather than wage-earning producers.

The discursive space, however, is just one arena of negotiation and resistance by the surrogates. Over the six years of my fieldwork, gradual shifts in the nature of resistances and negotiations became visible. As media coverage of the clinic and surrogacy increases, the stigma of surrogacy starts getting diluted, and women, especially the repeat surrogates, start negotiating higher payments and more support from their families and start demanding less interference by brokers. This gradual shift in the nature of resistances and negotiations—from the everyday mundane and symbolic acts of resistances to demands for changes in the actual labor market conditions—is a critical part of this story of commercial surrogacy in India.

INDIA: THE "MOTHER DESTINATION" FOR COMMERCIAL SURROGACY

See Taj Mahal by the moonlight while your embryo grows in a Petri-dish.
—A reproductive tourism website

Our pregnancy rates are very high, because we can transfer more embryos in difficult patients, unlike in UK and Australia.
—Rotunda Center for Human Reproduction

With PlanetHospital, all you have to do is show up.
—Planethospital.com

The Indian case represents an especially interesting site because India is the first country in the global south with a flourishing industry in national and transnational commercial surrogacy.[11] Although the United States remains the top global destination for commercial surrogacy, India is fast emerging as a key player, labeled by some as the "mother destination" for commercial gestational surrogacy (Rudrappa 2012). It is worth noting that almost all cases of commercial surrogacy in India, and all the cases in this study, are gestational rather than traditional. Gestational surrogacy is a variant of surrogacy in which the surrogate conceives using in vitro fertilization with the egg of the intended mother or an egg donor that has been fertilized in a petri dish with sperm provided by the intended father (or, in some cases, a donor). In traditional surrogacy, on the other hand, the surrogate provides the eggs as well as the womb. The intended parents, therefore, are more likely to emphasize the "right" genetic makeup, such as race, physical characteristics, and education of the surrogate. In gestational surrogacy, however, the surrogate's genetic makeup becomes less relevant for the client, since she theoretically provides only her womb. Not surprisingly, the gestational variant of surrogacy plays a critical role in the growing popularity of transnational surrogacy. India is not the only country to experience transnational surrogacy. Clients from countries where surrogacy is either illegal or restricted (such as Britain, Japan, Australia, Taiwan, and Kuwait) have hired surrogates in the United States to bear babies for them. But while the total cost of such transnational packages is roughly $100,000, in India the price is less than a third of that.[12]

What makes the Indian case all the more interesting is that the market is flourishing with very few formal regulations. Although commercial surrogacy is legal in India, there are currently no laws regulating the procedures, the contract, or the surrogate-client relationship. As a consequence, intended parents are able to take advantage of the client-friendly policies of private clinics and hospitals, where doctors are willing to offer options and services that are banned or heavily regulated in other parts of the world. Because of the moral and ethical ambiguity surrounding surrogacy, most countries treat commercial surrogacy with utmost caution. Some countries, like China, France, Germany, Italy, Saudi Arabia, Switzerland, Taiwan, and Turkey, have taken the prohibitive approach and banned surrogacy in all its forms. Some, including Australia (Victoria), Brazil, Canada, Hong Kong, Hungary, Mexico, South Africa, and the U.K., have imposed partial bans and allow altruistic surrogacy.[13] Even the United States, which usually takes a laissez-faire approach to most fertility treatments, is more cautious in the context of commercial surrogacy arrangements—surrogacy is regulated not by the federal government but through a combination of legislative actions and court decisions. This legal inconsistency among states means that clients may not be able to access surrogacy services in their own state and often travel to another, more surrogacy-friendly state, for instance California. The Indian structure is close to the liberal market model of surrogacy in California, and clinics can follow their own set of "informal rules." Clinics in India, however, not only operate without state interference but often benefit from explicit state support for clinics catering to medical and reproductive travelers. In 2004 the government launched an international advertising campaign and declared that treatment of foreign patients is legally an export and deemed eligible for all fiscal incentives extended to export earnings.[14]

There are other factors working in favor of India as a destination for such travel—cheap costs, large numbers of well-qualified and English-speaking doctors with degrees and training from prestigious medical schools in India and abroad, well-equipped private clinics, and a large overseas population of Indian origin who often combine cheaper treatment with a family visit. International clients are also drawn by the paucity of regulations and informality of contracts in India. Fertility clinics like Armaan (a pseudonym), the clinic that I studied, are free to take or reject the suggestions made by the National Guidelines for Accreditation, Supervision, and Regulation of ART Clinics in India issued by the Indian Council of Medical Research (ICMR) in 2005. In November 2010, the ICMR submitted a final set of guidelines for the ART Act (Assisted Reproductive Technologies) to the law ministry (see appendix A). In January 2013, the home ministry laid out another list of guidelines, or "clauses," that need to be followed if foreign nationals are to be issued a visa for surrogacy (Rajadhyaksha 2013). A clause that is likely to have a serious impact on the transnational market, especially the growing clientele of gay foreigners, is that only couples who have been married for two years and those whose countries recognize surrogacy can apply for a medical visa for surrogacy. But as of now (2013), clinics continue to work informally, and can, in effect, make or break their own rules. For instance, Armaan has its informal set of rules for recruiting surrogates: the woman should not be older than 40, should be medically fit, and should have a healthy uterus;

she should be married, with at least one healthy child; and, finally, she should have her husband's consent. The rules are much less stringent for clients: the client needs only to prove a history of infertility. In 2006 the clinic accepted only married heterosexual couples. But in 2008 the doctor had given in to the growing clientele of gay couples and single fathers and was accepting gay clients from all over the world. This is likely to be affected by the latest "clause" added to the existing guidelines, but it is still too early to speculate.[15]

Despite recent attempts by the Indian government to regulate the flow of international clients, the ICMR guidelines remain ambiguous and often misleading with regard to pertinent issues like the parentage and citizenship of babies born through surrogacy.[16] The inadequacies of the guidelines are revealed by the recent spate of custody and citizenship controversies surrounding surrogate births. The first of these was the much publicized "Baby Manji" case—an unusual kind of custody battle, with a biological father from Japan fighting for custody of a baby girl, a baby girl no one else really wanted ("Japanese Baby . . . " 2008). The couple from Japan had hired the services of a surrogate mother and used the eggs of an anonymous donor. Just a month before the baby was born, the couple separated. When his ex-wife refused to travel with him to take possession of the baby, the intended father flew to India alone. The Indian authorities, however, refused to give the baby to its father because the Guardian Wards Act of 1890 bans single men from adopting girls in India. The next few weeks saw the drama unfold with a weeping grandmother making her appearance from Japan to convince authorities that they should give her custody of her granddaughter, Manji. Manji was being declared the first surrogate orphan. Ultimately there was a happy ending, with the Indian Supreme Court stepping in and directing the government to give Manji a travel certificate for Japan. The second, more recent "surrogacy orphan" case involved an intended mother from the United States, an intended father from Jamaica, and a baby carried by a surrogate in India using the eggs of an anonymous Indian donor. The intended mother "caused a flutter" at the passport office when she abandoned the baby in protest against the delay in issuing a passport to the child ("U.S. Woman . . . " 2012). The case generated much media debate about the legal lacunae surrounding citizenship of such babies.

But not all surrogacy battles get such media attention. The most sobering, yet least publicized, were two cases in which the surrogates died as a result of birth-related complications. In 2009, a young surrogate started suffering from uncontrollable bleeding just a few days after delivering the baby. The clinic, unprepared for complications, told her husband to book his own ambulance to a nearby hospital. The woman died on the way to the hospital. Not surprisingly, neither the clinic nor the intended parents were ready to take responsibility for the young woman's death (Carney 2010). In a similar case in 2012, a surrogate collapsed due to "unexplained complications" in the eighth month of her pregnancy. The clinic was able to perform an emergency surgery and save the baby. According to media reports, the surrogate "completed her job," delivered the baby to the American couple, and died soon after ("Surrogate Mother Dies . . . " 2012). But in 2006, when my journey began, the surrogacy scandals were yet to unfold.

"PARTICIPANT" OBSERVATION? DILEMMAS OF A FEMINIST ETHNOGRAPHER

When I started my research in 2006, surrogacy was in its nascent stages in India, and there had been only ten births at the clinic. It was not just the small number of cases that posed a challenge. Although surrogacy is shrouded in secrecy in almost all countries, surrogates are unusually stigmatized in India. This is partly because many Indians equate surrogacy with sex work. People are not aware of the reproductive technology aspect of surrogacy that separates pregnancy from sexual intercourse. The popular media, including movies and television shows, add to this misconception by equating surrogates with sex workers. Perhaps because of the secrecy, my field trip was bumpy at the outset. The main doctor and proprietor of Armaan clinic, Dr. Khanderia (a pseudonym), was unexpectedly welcoming in her first few e-mail messages. But two days before my departure from Boston she changed her mind. "Please do not come here. No one wants to speak to you." Needless to say, I was devastated. I decided, however, to take a risk and forge ahead. Fortunately, my impetuosity did not backfire. Over my years of fieldwork, the surrogates, the nurses, and even the brokers not only gave consent willingly, but some of them did not stop talking even when the tape recorder ran out of power.

Being a woman from India gave me many advantages in the field. Many of the surrogates spoke freely about contraceptives and the bodily effects of surrogacy. While my education and "recent U.S. return" status were causes for much admiration, my then unmarried status generated a lot of sympathy. The women often patted me on my back and reassured me that my "chance" (to get married) would come soon. My single status and unfamiliarity with their customs made them treat me like a younger person who needed assistance—although most of the women were either my age or younger. Despite the camaraderie and the apparent ease with which I fit into the surrogacy hostel, the class difference between us was always apparent. My tape recorder, my bottle of mineral water, and my incessant scribbling on a notepad set me apart as the strange, educated woman from the United States. Throughout my fieldwork this insider-outsider identity remained a dilemma. On the one hand, I did not want to be an outsider and make the surrogates feel either intimidated or alienated. On the other hand, I did not want to fit in too well either. Most of the women had kept their surrogacy a secret from their community and were reluctant to talk to local media. My ambiguous identity was reassuring for the women, and they spoke to me openly about issues they seldom mentioned to journalists.

In spite of the relationship that I established with the surrogates, I was aware that many agreed to give the initial consent because of the doctor's request. The doctor and the nurses introduced me to my first round of respondents—surrogates in the clinic. Thereafter, the surrogates referred me to their friends, families, brokers, and other women who had already delivered. This awareness made me even more cautious about maintaining the surrogates' privacy; I refrained from taking photographs (unless the surrogates wanted me to take photographs with them), and I got their consent before starting any recorded conversation. Some surrogates refused to give me their real names, while some did not want me to record our conversations. Then there were others who insisted on being recorded and even got offended if I recorded their friends' narratives and took only handwritten notes on their comments. They often reminded me to switch my recorder on, and some asked me to rewind the tape so they could hear how they sounded and review what they had said. I tape-recorded most conversations. In the cases where respondents felt uncomfortable having their narratives recorded, I took extensive handwritten notes that I typed immediately afterward. Over the course of time, most surrogates not only talked to me willingly, but often asked me to sit by their bedside and then started telling me their life experiences without any prompting. Most felt reassured when I told them that I was not from any Indian television company or local newspaper. One of my informants, Rita, echoed the sentiment of many others when she told

Regina (another surrogate at the clinic), "This poor girl, she needs to fill up her whole notepad before she can make a book out of it. We should all talk as much as we can and help her do it as quickly as possible."

I have used pseudonyms for the names of all places and people. Garv is a pseudonym for the city that has emerged as the surrogacy center in India, and Armaan is the pseudonym for the clinic. I used real names in only four cases, since those surrogates asked me to use their real names. Some of the surrogates found the concept of using pseudonyms very amusing, and often the first few minutes of our conversations were spent giggling over an appropriate pseudonym for them.

This book is based on fieldwork conducted between 2006 and 2011. My research has included in-depth, open-format interviews with 52 surrogates, their husbands and in-laws, 12 intending parents, three doctors, three surrogacy brokers, three hostel matrons, and several nurses. In the first two years of fieldwork, I conducted interviews with 42 surrogates, the husbands of 28 surrogates and the in-laws of 18 surrogates, eight intended parents, two doctors, and two surrogacy brokers. Typically, the interviews with surrogates were unstructured, with my opening question being: "Tell me your life story from wherever you feel important and also how you got involved in this process." The interviews with their families and the medical staff were more structured in nature. All the interviews were conducted in Hindi and the local language of the region, ranged from one hour to five hours in length, and were conducted at the clinic, at the hostels where most surrogates live, or at their homes. Apart from the interviews, I conducted participant observation for more than nine months at the surrogacy clinic and two surrogacy hostels. What typically distinguishes participant observation is that the researcher studies people in their own time and space, in their everyday lives, as opposed to in the unnatural setting of the interview or the laboratory (Burawoy 1991). It has been argued that the advantages of participant observation lie not just in direct observation of how people act but also in how they understand and experience those acts. But these virtues can become dangers whereby the intimacy of the researcher's relationship with the participants in her research work can allegedly lead to "loss of objectivity" or to "contamination" of the situation (1991, 2). I recognize that my intimate relationship with the surrogates often blurred the boundary between formal research and the everyday. During my fieldwork I engaged in formal research activities like conducting interviews with the doctors and surrogacy brokers, preparing questionnaires for nurses and brokers, and collecting demographic information on the area from local libraries. But I also had lunches and teas with the surrogates and their families, smuggled in tea-time snacks for surrogates, prayed and cooked lunches for them in the surrogacy hostel. After months of constant interactions with the surrogates I found myself immersed in the intricacies of their lives and felt torn between my roles as a researcher and as a friend. I wanted to intervene when the nurses left out important information about side effects of some injections, when they gave minimal details to the (often illiterate) surrogates, or treated them callously. But in spite of the relationship I established with the surrogates, I could not openly voice my opinion. My presence at the clinic depended on the doctor's and the hostel matron's consent. I initially tried not to immerse myself in the working of the clinic and the surrogate community, but ultimately immersion became the source of the richest and the most invaluable conversations and experiences.

This immersion became even deeper when I had an unexpected opportunity to revisit the surrogacy hostels yet again in 2011. Ditte Maria Bjerg, a Danish feminist stage director and artistic director of Global Stories, a social theater group based in Denmark, approached me to collaborate with her on a theater production on commercial surrogacy as well as to facilitate a livelihood-generating workshop with the surrogates.[17] I was, at that time, in my sixth month of pregnancy and unsure as to how my pregnancy would be perceived by the surrogates themselves. My concerns about potentially being a disrespectful researcher were dismissed in no uncertain terms by the former surrogates and friends whom I contacted via e-mail and telephone. The former and repeat surrogates were eager to celebrate the "naive" researcher in her new avatar. My new status as a married and pregnant woman generated lively discussions on motherhood, bodily changes, emotional upheavals, labor pains, and marital relationships—topics that the women were reluctant to discuss with me when I was unmarried and hence, in their words, naive and inexperienced. My pregnancy was celebrated enthusiastically by the women, but it inadvertently highlighted the poignancy of their "surrogate" pregnancies. The women's response to the difference between our pregnancies and their spontaneous reflections on alienation of labor, among other things, are discussed in the empirical chapters of the book. This journey also gave me the opportunity to interview 10 more surrogates and revisit five surrogates I had interviewed in 2006—three of the five women had been surrogates more than once, and two were pregnant (for the third time) and at the hostel during my visit in 2011. I conducted an impromptu group discussion with these "veteran" surrogates. Their reflections on various aspects of the surrogacy industry over the years are analyzed in the epilogue.

SURROGATES AT ARMAAN

In March 2013 Armaan clinic announced the birth of the 500th baby through surrogacy. By December 2013, the clinic was getting ready to celebrate the birth of the 600th baby. More than 300 surrogates had been matched with couples from India and from 29 other countries, including the United States, Japan, South Africa, the United Kingdom, and Spain. While the wide range of international clients makes Armaan clinic exceptionally newsworthy, the demography of its surrogates makes it controversial. Simply put, surrogates in this study, and most surrogates at the clinic, are poorer than their counterparts in other known studies of surrogacy. In her study of global surrogacy, France Winddance Twine suggests that the "majority of women who provide gestational service are poor or members of racial or ethnic minority groups" (2011, 9). To my knowledge, there are no nationwide data on the economic profile of surrogates in the United States. However, Twine's systematic comparison of the wages of a typical gestational surrogate in the United States to women working in other industries (like retail sales and nursing) seems to indicate that surrogacy may well be an appealing alternative for women who are not necessarily economically desperate. In addition, since surrogates also get health insurance, medical benefits, and a monthly stipend, Twine concludes that surrogacy may well be an "attractive alternative to working in jobs that provide comparable wages" (19). Another news report on surrogacy in the United States indicates that military wives in the United States who decide to become surrogates can potentially earn three times their husbands' annual salary (Ali and Kelley 2008). It is also likely that since some U.S. surrogacy programs reject women if they are not financially stable, desperately poor women are not able to choose this "appealing alternative." In Elly Teman's (2010) study of surrogacy in Israel, surrogates were more upfront about their financial needs, and most accepted that they were in surrogacy to supplement their income. Although many surrogates were single mothers struggling to support their children, only 20 percent of Teman's interviewees could be classified as desperately poor (24).

In sharp contrast to the above cases, all but one of the surrogates at Armaan reported acute financial desperation. The median family income of surrogates was about $50 per month in 2006. If we compare that to the official poverty line (approximately $10 per person per month for rural areas and approximately $13 a month for urban areas), 36 of my interviewees reported a family income that put them below the poverty line (Planning Commission of India 2012). For most of the surrogates' families, the money earned through surrogacy was equivalent to approximately five years of total family income, especially since many had husbands who were either in informal contract work or unemployed. Most of the women were driven to surrogacy because of financial desperation, often compounded by a medical emergency and an urgent need for liquid cash. Although some recent reports have hinted that "middle-class" women too are becoming surrogates in other clinics (Cohen 2009; Rudrappa 2012), only two women identified as middle class in my six years of fieldwork.[18] All the surrogates in this study were married, with at least one child. The ages of the surrogates ranged between 20 and 45 years. Except for two surrogates, all the women were from neighboring villages. Fourteen of the women said that they were "housewives," two said they "worked at home," and the others worked at schools, clinics, farms, and stores. Their education ranged from illiterate to high school level, with the average being a middle-school level. Transnational clients had hired 30 of the respondents (see table 1).

MAPPING THE BOOK

The recent spurt of international custody battles has put surrogacy in India in the spotlight, and earlier predictions of baby farms and breeding factories are starting to resurface. Being one of the first to research extensively on a so-called "sensational" topic is as challenging as it is exhilarating. It is not my intention in this book to depict surrogates in India as breeders or clinics in India as baby farms. On the contrary, I caution against such speculations and potentially orientalist frames for understanding the impact of new reproductive technologies on women of the global south. Instead, I use my sustained interactions with the surrogates, medical staff, and clients, as well as my observation of the industry in Garv, to reveal the workings of this labor market and the way the various actors experience it. This book is meant for scholars of reproduction, reproductive technology, globalization, and gendered forms of labor, but it is also intended for anyone who is interested in understanding the workings of this booming national and transnational industry. This introductory chapter sets the stage by describing the field and providing an analysis of existing debates on assisted reproductive technology.

In chapter 2, "Pro-natal Technologies in an Anti-natal State," I provide a brief sketch of the contradictory history of the rise and spread of surrogacy in India. Historically, the Indian state is aggressively anti-natalist, and despite ostensible changes in population policies over time, the sterilization of women, especially young, lower-class women, remains the mainstay of these policies. This nationalist ideal of "population control" along with international pressures for economic liberalization has led to two contradictory trends—a retreat by the state as a healthcare provider for the poor but an enthusiastic embrace by the state as an advocate of medical tourism and private investment in biotechnologies for the rich. Moreover, cultural and economic restrictions have meant that medicalization of childbirth has historically remained relatively low in most parts of India and hospital births are still not the norm. Most surrogates in my study have never had the opportunity to benefit from professionalized medical care, and the hyper-medicalized surveillance of commercial surrogacy was often their first encounter with medicalized birth and health care. A critical analysis of this history reveals the different layers of domination faced by the surrogate—from the family, the clinic, and the state. But a familiarity with this history is also vital to appreciate the negotiations of these layers of domination by the surrogates, an aspect that is explored in later chapters.

Chapter 3, "When the Fish Talk About the Water," introduces readers to the surrogates as they describe their initiation into the surrogacy process. These narratives provide insight on their involvement and their awareness about the surrogacy processes, the contract, and payment, as well as their experience of surrogacy before the actual delivery. In the epilogue I contrast these expectations to evaluations of the surrogacy experience *after* the delivery. Did a surrogate's initiation into surrogacy determine her overall experiences of surrogacy? Do women who choose surrogacy have more control over their earnings than women who are pushed into it by brokers or family members? One might assume that women who *choose* surrogacy as an option—relatively educated women and women who have previously been employed outside of the house—are likely to benefit most from this labor option and are also likely have more control over the earnings. In this chapter I examine trends in recruitment to demystify many of these assumptions.

Recruiting a surrogate is just one step in the surrogacy process. In chapter 4, "Manufacturing the Perfect Mother-Worker," I argue that a perfect commercial surrogate is not found ready-made but is actively *produced* in fertility clinics and surrogacy hostels. Surrogacy is remarkable as a form of labor in the way it requires the laborer to be both a mother and a worker. The disciplinary project exploits this duality in intriguing ways. The surrogate is expected to be a disciplined contract worker who gives up the baby at the termination of the contract. But she is simultaneously urged to be a nurturing mother for the baby, and a selfless mother who will not negotiate the payment received. When one's identity as a mother is regulated and terminated by a contract, being a good mother often conflicts with being a good worker, which makes the disciplinary project not just contradictory but also particularly repressive. It works discursively, through language and metaphor, and physically in the form of dormitory-like surrogacy hostels. The surrogacy contract and counseling produce a perfect mother-worker "mind"—the surrogate is constructed as a disposable and somewhat dirty worker, as well as a disposable mother with no real ties to the baby. Meanwhile, the surrogacy hostel with its active partitioning of space and time disciplines the surrogate's body. And through the various stages the perfect "mother-worker" for national and international clients is produced.

In chapter 5, "Everyday Divinities and God's Labor," I demonstrate how the disciplinary project shapes the interplay of divinity and surrogacy in the narratives of the surrogates themselves. An underlying tactic of the disciplinary project, the counseling, and the contract is to mystify the process of surrogacy. Most surrogates do not understand what surrogacy really entails, and this unfamiliar, unexplained technology takes the shape of the "divine." I demonstrate that for surrogates at Armaan clinic and hostel, "everyday divine" takes precedence over organized religion. The process of surrogacy and the doctor herself are deified, while religious endogamy and prescriptions are underplayed. But apart from constructing such creative forms of divinity, the narratives of divinity are startling on another front. Previous ethnographies of surrogacy in other parts of the world have revealed that surrogates often construct the surrogate birth as their divine gift to the commissioning parents, and themselves as angels and messengers of God (Teman 2010). The disciplined surrogates of India, however, construct surrogacy as God's gift to needy and poor Indian mothers. The idioms of "God's labor," "mission," and "angel" are instead evoked by the doctors, brokers, and intended mothers. In the narratives of these other women, surrogates are constructed as the worthy poor, and the payment is constructed as donation toward a "worthy cause." In essence, such narratives of the divine reify the disciplinary project; the good surrogate hesitates to negotiate the payment and instead treats it as God's gift to her to fulfill her familial responsibilities.

One of the most unusual aspects of surrogacy as labor is its extreme corporality: the resources, the skills, and the ultimate product are derived primarily from the body of the laborer. The body is central, and hence the body is monitored, disciplined, and controlled. Chapter 6, "Embodied Labor and Neo-eugenics," introduces the reader not just to the bodily requirements and bodily effects of surrogacy in India, but also to the body as a space of resistance. I use the term "embodied labor," a form of labor that involves a rental of one's body by somebody else, in which the body of the worker is the fundamental and ultimate site, resource, requirement, and (arguably) its product, to analyze the surrogates' response to the disciplinary project outlined in chapter 4. As the hyper-medicalized body of the surrogate comes under increased scrutiny, the surrogates reclaim control over their bodies by using their bodies for labor. To do this, the surrogates negotiate with not just the clinic but also their families, especially their husbands and in-laws. But these individual resistances have unintended consequences, and challenges to one form of domination almost inevitably lead to reification of another. I expand on Shellee Colen's (1995) notion of "stratified reproduction" and Dorothy Roberts's (1997) conceptualization of the race-based reproductive hierarchy, to argue that surrogacy in India is an explicit manifestation of "neo-eugenics." This is the new, subtle form of eugenics whereby the neoliberal notion of consumer choice justifies promotion of assisted reproductive services for the rich and, at the same time, justifies aggressive anti-natal policies by portraying poor people (often in the global south) as strains on the world's economy and environment. Moreover, as the surrogates align their own reproduction, through decisions about fertility, sterilization, and abortion, in order to (re)produce children of higher classes and privileged nations, they ultimately conform to this neoliberal global imperative of reducing the fertility of lower-class women in the global south.

The body of the surrogate is just one part of the disciplinary project, and correspondingly just one avenue for the surrogates to negotiate, resist, and subvert. Equally critical to the disciplinary project is the production of the perfect mother-worker mind. In chapter 7, "Disposable Workers and Dirty Labor," I analyze how the surrogates negotiate the stigmatizing labels of being disposable and dirty workers. From recruitment to delivery, the surrogate-whore comparison plays a critical role in the disciplinary project. It is simultaneously challenged and reinforced by the brokers, counselors, and medical professionals at different stages of the labor process. The surrogate stigma stems not only from the disciplinary project but also from the broader understanding of surrogacy external to the clinic. Like the whore stigma, the surrogate stigma reflects deeply felt anxieties about women trespassing the dangerous boundaries between the private and the public. Selling wombs for pay becomes an anomaly, much like selling bodies for pay. The high level of stigma attached to surrogacy in India brings out fascinating parallels between commercial surrogacy and other forms of "dirty labor"—work that is considered physically or morally degrading. The surrogates not only neutralize the stigma attached to this new form of dirty labor, but they tacitly, creatively, and sometimes explicitly contest other subject positions assigned to them by their families and community. But while the language of morality used by the surrogates resists the medical framing of surrogates as "disposable and dirty workers," it reinforces the gendered image of women as selfless, dutiful mothers whose primary role is to serve the family. Moreover, the dream of a wealthier family coming to rescue them from desperate poverty and a bleak future brings in issues of new forms of subjection based on race and class domination. The (often fictive) relationships formed with intended parents downplay the contractual and business aspect of surrogacy and further undermine the surrogates' ability to view themselves as workers and to defend their interests as such.

In chapter 8, "Disposable Mothers and Kin Labor," I introduce the concept of "kin labor," a subversive strategy used by the surrogates to challenge the medical construction of surrogates as "disposable mothers." Surrogates respond to the medical construction of surrogates as disposable mothers by forging kin ties with the baby, the intended mother, and other surrogates living in the hostel. The surrogates' constructions of kinship denaturalize kin ties by highlighting labor as a basis for making kinship claims. This includes not just the labor of gestation and giving birth but also the kin labor (sending gifts, writing letters, and keeping in touch even after the delivery of the baby) done by surrogates with one another and with the intended mothers. These new and creative bases of kin ties disrupt the construction of Indian kinship as a bounded sphere constrained by not just patriliny but also interactions within the same caste and religion. Once again I highlight the poignancy of these subversive strategies and the kin ties. The surrogates form kin ties that disrupt the sanctity of biology and genes within a system that might well be the pinnacle of the commodification of the genetic tie. The alleged "beauty" of gestational surrogacy, relative to traditional surrogacy or transnational adoption, is that the hiring couple need not cross any borders and that the child carries its parents' genes. In the end, the surrogates' claims of kinship do not prevent the clinic from taking the baby away from them—usually immediately after birth.

In the concluding section, I bring together the many paradoxes of surrogacy revealed in the book. In order to speculate about future policy options, I evaluate the paradoxical nature of surrogacy in general as well as concerns specific to the form that commercial surrogacy takes in India. I lay out for the readers the implications of two possible choices: an outright ban (national or transnational) on surrogacy or a regulatory framework. I argue that the former is not just unfeasible but also undesirable in the Indian context. Instead of a ban, I advocate for a better understanding of this complex labor market and subsequently its transformation through policies based on the real lived experiences of the surrogates as revealed in this book. Finally I argue that a global issue like transnational surrogacy cannot be dealt with nationally and regulations cannot preclude international awareness and dialogue. I connect some recent insights on "fair trade international surrogacy" to my ethnographic findings and advocate for an international model of surrogacy founded on openness and transparency on three fronts: in the medical process, in the payments made to the different actors involved in surrogacy, and in the relationships forged within surrogacy.

The national and international media, the doctors, and the intended parents unanimously claim that surrogacy magically transforms the lives of families living in desperate poverty in India. By revisiting previously interviewed women after their delivery, the epilogue—"Did the 'Sperm on a Rickshaw' Save the Third World?"—asks a simple question: do the lives of surrogates, in fact, get transformed? I analyze the real and diverse impact of surrogacy on the lives of surrogates: how surrogacy affects their livelihood, their families, and the gendered division of labor, as well as their attitudes toward work and motherhood.

2 ◢ PRO-NATAL TECHNOLOGIES
IN AN ANTI-NATAL STATE

*Women of the South . . . are increasingly reduced to numbers, targets, wombs, tubes
and other reproductive parts by the population controllers.*

—Maria Mies and Vandana Shiva, *Ecofeminism*

*Women live at once under the scrutiny of the state and transnational forces of inter-
vention and at a remove from the certainties of life captured in the term "infrastructure" or the fantasy of "health care."*

—Sarah Pinto, *Where There Is No Midwife*

A DETAILED ACCOUNT of the social history of India is not plausible
here. What is necessary, however, is a brief sketch of the strangely
contradictory history of the landscape that forms the context for
the rise and spread of surrogacy. How does a labor market based on pro-
natal technologies fit in the context of an aggressively anti-natalist state?
How do we analyze the sudden hyper-medicalization of childbirth for a
group of women previously exposed to very low rates of medicalization?

MEDICALIZATION OF CHILDBIRTH

Critiques of the Western biomedical model of birth have argued that "technological interventions serve primarily to shift control over the birth process from the mother to the (often male) doctor" (Van Hollen 2003, 51). This
argument emerges from a specific sociocultural context and can be traced
back to the Enlightenment era, where female midwives gradually came
to be replaced by male doctors (Anderson and Bauwens 1982; Davis-Floyd

1990; Van Hollen 2003). Pregnant women were constructed as "potentially pathological" and as "patients" who needed constant surveillance (Van Hollen 2003, 50). In response, feminist activists resisted the biomedicalization and professionalization of childbirth in the United States and Europe by advocating a return to natural childbirth and to women-centered home births attended by female midwives. However, as reproductive processes become increasingly biomedicalized across the globe, we cannot assume that this process occurs in a uniform way (Lock and Kaufert 2000).[1] For India, the two differences that stand out in particular are, first, the historically low rate of medicalization and professionalization of childbirth, and second, the high level of state surveillance of childbirth and fertility.

In the late nineteenth and early twentieth centuries, the "management of childbirth emerged as a key issue in colonial and nationalist discourses in India." The growing interest in maternal and infant mortality was partly the result of "pronatalist fears of depopulation" and colonial anxiety about a "shrinking labor pool" in the colony (Van Hollen 2003, 36). The colonial state's "concern" for maternal and infant mortality was partly also designed to legitimize colonialism as necessary for the emancipation of the vulnerable subaltern women. The state thus promoted professionalization of obstetrics as the solution to the problem of high mortality during childbirth. Despite these early attempts by the colonial state, medicalization of childbirth remained relatively low in most parts of India, and hospital births did not become (and still are not) the norm in India.[2]

As can be expected, issues of class, rural/urban residence, and caste also influenced the ways in which birth gradually become professionalized in India. For instance, "cultural restrictions against women being examined or touched by a male doctor, especially during childbirth, meant that one could find many more female obstetricians in India during the early history of obstetrics than in Europe and the United States" (Van Hollen 2003, 53). In the late nineteenth century, for instance, there were hospitals called "*Zanana* hospitals," reserved for women and run by female nurses (Mavalankar and Vora 2008). Another critical factor shaping biomedicalization is place of residence. There is a definite rural-urban differential in healthcare utilization, with women in rural areas utilizing health care at lower levels than their urban counterparts (Mistry, Galal, and Lu 2009). In rural India, trained professionals or auxiliary nurse midwives (ANMs) are expected to interact directly with the community and provide basic medical care (Mavalankar and Vora 2008). A majority of reproductive services is ostensibly provided by these ANMs. In theory, the

ANMs are expected to "provide a variety of regular services to pregnant women"—medical checkups, distribution of essential medicines and vitamins, administration of injections—as well as to assist in their deliveries whenever required (Shariff and Singh 2002, 11). But over the years, the focus of ANMs has undergone a shift from basic community health and delivery services to targeted family planning (Mavalankar and Vora 2008). The ANMs are also expected to maintain a network of *dais* (midwives), with some basic training in home delivery (Shariff and Singh 2002). But in practice, as a result of corruption and/or inadequate support systems, dais seldom establish contact with pregnant women. Arguably, the low utilization of institutional delivery services is not only a result of limited access. Even when professional nurses or dais are available, women in rural areas rarely consult them during pregnancy. Pregnancy, in general, is "looked upon as a condition that does not require medical attention" (Shariff and Singh 2002, 12). Home delivery is preferred to institutional delivery, especially in large multigeneration families where the older women can provide traditional maternity and childbirth information and advice as well as assistance at the time of delivery (Munjial, Kaushik, and Agnihotri 2009; Shariff and Singh 2002).

Significant differences exist in the demographic, regional, and economic profiles of the users and the non-users of reproductive healthcare services (Ahmed and Mosley 1997; Das, Mishra, and Saha 2001; Govindasamy 2000; Hazarika 2010; Kanitkar and Sinha 1989). Home births are more likely in rural India, where nearly three-quarters of all births continue to take place at home without any involvement by trained professionals (Mishra and Retherford 2008). Other studies have reported the low utilization of institutionalized delivery facilities by women in urban slums (Agrawal and Bharti 2006; Hazarika 2010; Mony et al. 2006).[3] Education (of the woman and her husband) increases the use of prenatal and postnatal care, as well as the use of skilled help at the time of delivery, and decreases the probability of a home delivery (Das, Mishra, and Saha 2001; Govindasamy and Ramesh 1997; Hazarika 2010). Although households with higher income are less likely to choose home delivery and more likely to use trained help for delivery, income alone does not seem to affect the use of prenatal and postnatal care. In fact, in rural areas, women from rich land- and business-owning households are less likely to use prenatal and postnatal care than those from the landless agricultural labor class. In rural India, cultural and traditional practices often "isolate pregnant women and restrict their physical movements" (Shariff and Singh 2002, 33). These practices are more likely to be observed in the landed and upper caste/class house-holds, restricting the healthcare access of women in these households despite their ability to afford such care (Shariff 1993; Shariff and Singh 2002). Other factors that affect the use of prenatal and postnatal care are the caste and religion of the household. Muslim women and those from what are labeled the "schedule caste and tribes" use significantly less pre-natal and postnatal care than upper-caste Hindu women (Navaneetham and Dharmalingam 2002; Saroha, Altarac, and Sibley 2008; Shariff 1993; Shariff and Singh 2002).

But apart from these factors at the local level, one of the most "signifi-cant factors influencing women's experiences of childbirth in the post-colonial era has been the (international and national) developmentalist agenda of population control" (Van Hollen 2003, 53).

"FAMILY PLANNING" AND THE SURVEILLANCE OF REPRODUCTION

Some of the earliest debates around birth control can be traced back to the early twentieth-century anti-natalist campaigns in India. These campaigns were spearheaded by the Indian elite who believed that in modern India fecundity had to be restrained and rationalized (Jolly and Ram 2001). This focus on "birth control" as an indicator of modernity is not limited to India but has been evident among modernization theorists, policymakers, and planners across the world. Although there is "considerable debate over whether population growth rates actually hinder economic growth," a pop-ular assumption is that fertility control is an essential aspect of modern-ization (Chatterjee and Riley 2001, 817). But these fertility-control-driven modernization campaigns in India cannot be understood in isolation from similar movements in Britain and the United States. In her work on the history of birth control in colonial India from 1871 to 1946, feminist his-torian Sanjam Ahluwalia (2003) describes these "interconnected histories" as a "dialogue between Indian birth control activists and their British and American counterparts," like Margaret Sanger and Marie Stopes. This dia-logue, she argues, enables us to "understand the interconnected workings of power locally, nationally, and globally" (188). While people like Sanger and Stopes saw in India both a profitable market for their contraceptive tech-nologies and "a site for greater publicity and acceptance for their project," Indian advocates found in the international community a "support base for their politics" (Ahluwalia 2003, 191). These dialogues and connections among Indian and international reformers and the determined focus on birth control as a sign of modernity and rationality inevitably constructed the subaltern woman (especially those from the lower classes, lower castes, and Muslims) as backward, sexually irresponsible, and immoral.

The Indian woman was the primary target of nationalist reformist agendas such as the population control campaigns partly because "archaic" practices like sati (suttee), child marriage, and polygamy had been used by British colonizers to legitimize their civilizing mission. But "modernity" needed to be defined cautiously. The modern Indian woman had to be distinguished not only from the archaic woman but also from the Westernized, "individualistic" woman. This is what Nilanjana Chatterjee and Nancy E. Riley (2001) call the "the nationalist leadership's selective appropriation of modernity" (819). For instance, nationalist reformers and activists supported the use of contraception for improving maternal and child health and not as a means to greater female autonomy. Autonomy was seen as a "distinctly Western notion and therefore not necessarily desirable" (821). This continues to be the underlying philosophy of the government's agenda, which frames its anti-natalist policy as "family welfare planning." Such framing avoids the association of contraceptive use with so-called Western notions of sexual freedom and "autonomy" and at the same time reaffirms the state's initiative in "upholding the traditional institution of the family" (Chatterjee and Riley 2001, 836). Regardless of the jargon used for state policies, the underlying impact of this anti-natalist ambition has been state surveillance of fertility, especially of poor and working-class women.

The most fundamental difference between state policies in many countries in the global north and in India is that unlike in the global north, where many women historically had to struggle to get access to the most basic birth control methods, in India the state forced it on them (Hartmann 1995). This is what Sarah Pinto (2008) astutely labels the "irony of eroded choice": the obsessive attention that the state pays to population control, often at the cost of broader health services, erodes the very notion of choice or democracy that ostensibly underlies such policies (18). In 1952 the Indian state became the first in the world to initiate an official population program. Unlike China, the democratic state of India had to maintain its liberal stance, but in reality these "liberal principles were constantly eroded by numerical targets, financial (dis)incentives, and sometimes aggressive promotion of sterilization" (Jolly and Ram 2001, 22). For instance, the political defeat suffered by the Indira Gandhi–led Congress in 1977 was attributed for the most part to the forced sterilizations of men between 1975 and 1977—the years of the National Emergency.[4] In general, the sterilization program was implemented with coercion and, not surprisingly, the illiterate, economically disadvantaged, scheduled castes and Muslims were the primary targets (Karkal 1998). Although the period of national emergency is remembered and criticized mostly for the forced sterilizations of men, it was also the time when many questionable methods of birth control were being aggressively propagated. These included IUDs, long-acting hormone-based contraception, such as Net-En, Depo-Provera, Norplant, and anti-fertility vaccines.[5] It is worth noting that a 19-month state "emergency" program forcing sterilization of *men* could mobilize enough widespread protest to overthrow a political party in power. Forced sterilization of women (under different garb) for two decades prior to that could not generate as much mass mobilizing. Despite the "illusion" that a democratic state offers every contraceptive choice to its citizens, in fact almost from its inception the Indian state has typically promoted methods that diminish women's power to choose— methods like sterilization and hormonal implants (Ram 2001, 90).

While sterilization was the highlight of the family planning program in India in the 1970s and 1980s, more recently the government has started advocating a voluntary two-child norm. The two-child norm "encourages" couples to adopt a permanent method after their second child, with disincentives for those who do not comply with this norm. For instance, in 2003 the Supreme Court of India upheld the rights of individual states to make the two-child norm a precondition for elected representatives (Das 2003). Several state governments have listed a series of incentives— educational concessions, subsidies, and promotions in as well as recruitment to government jobs—for those adhering to the small-family norm. Others offer consumer products, like motorcycles, TV sets, or mixer-grinders, to people who accept sterilization, in an attempt to get top position in the race for sterilization drives (Ali 2011). Disincentives include barring women with more than two children from contesting elections, linking health insurance benefits to sterilization, and a proposal to deny food rations and free education to the third child (Visaria 2002; Visaria, Acharya, and Raj 2006).

The Indian population control program, however, cannot be discussed as just a nationalist agenda and cannot be understood without reference to the postwar international population movement dominated by governments and academicians from the global north. This population movement was shaped by a group of public and private organizations that included the Rockefeller Foundation, the Population Council, the United States Agency for International Development (USAID), the United Nations Population Fund (UNFPA), and the World Bank. These organizations invested not only in fertility control programs in countries like India but also in the training of administrators and students in these countries (Chatterjee and Riley 2001, 812). "The greatest foreign involvement in India's population agenda, however, came after the drought and the economic crisis of 1966 when India was pressured by the World Bank to intensify fertility reduction efforts along with a move toward economic liberalization" (Chatterjee and Riley 2001, 824). As a response, the government transformed the family planning program from a program providing voluntary services into an incentive and target-driven population reduction program.

The international pressures for economic liberalization not only resulted in an aggressive population control program but also meant a further retreat of the state as a provider of services, including health-care services. The state abandoned its earlier attempts at building a welfare state and accepted the structural adjustment program and policies (SAP). The SAP-mandated health sector reforms included cutbacks, withdrawal from the public sector, and opening up the sector to private investments and international capital.[6] In fact, government expenditure on public health infrastructure continues to remain as low as one percent of its gross domestic product, lower than the average of 2.8 percent of GDP spent by most less-developed countries ("Concern Over Draft Health Chapter . . . " 2012). Despite cuts in most areas of public expenditure, the government's budget for family planning has continued to increase.

Historically and globally, "the development of modern contraceptives and reproductive technologies has been gender asymmetrical," designed almost exclusively for women's bodies. With the exception of condoms and vasectomies, modern contraceptive technologies all over the world (the pill, the diaphragm, IUDs, tubal ligations, Depo-Provera, and Norplant) impact women's bodies (Jolly and Ram 2001, 25). But the development of modern contraceptives in India has asymmetries based on not just gender but also *class*. Right from the outset, "there was very little information disseminated about the contraceptive pill," which was seen as a "technology appropriate only for women in the global north and for upper-class, educated women in India" (22). Narayana and Kantner (1992) comment on the conviction among many government officials and family planning professionals that the "requirements of the pill regimen were beyond the powers of mind and discipline of illiterate Indian housewives" (111). The lower-class female consumer in state discourse was assumed to be someone who was recklessly fertile, someone "who could not be trusted" to not have babies (Jolly and Ram 2001, 22). This has a profound influence on women's interactions with government hospitals and public maternity wards, because these institutions, which are the primary source of health care for poorer communities, are a key arena within which the government tries to implement its birth control campaigns (Van Hollen 2003). Public healthcare systems are where women face intense pressure to undergo sterilization or accept IUDs immediately after birth (Jolly and Ram 2001; Van Hollen 1998, 2003). Poor women from rural areas are often reluctant to seek prenatal or postnatal care because of these pressures in public healthcare institutions. This fear and subsequent reluctance to seek public health care are compounded for women who are most marginalized—for instance, lower-caste and Muslim women (Pinto 2008).

The state's implicit attempts at eugenics—controlling the composition of the population by discouraging the reproductive potential of certain "undesirable groups" (namely the poor, the uneducated, and the rural)— are reflected not only in its policies but also in the consequences of these policies for different groups of women. For instance, studies indicate that women who have not finished middle school are far more likely than high school graduates to be sterilized (Remez 2001) and that use of reversible methods is significantly higher among better-educated women and those who rely on the private sector for their contraceptive needs. Illiterate and uneducated women from poor and landless rural backgrounds have the highest chances of getting sterilized. This is partly because they are not made aware of other reversible methods of contraception.

These structural disparities are, however, not restricted to technologies that *prevent* birth. In her work on the intersection of race, class, and the use of reproductive technologies in the United States, Dorothy Roberts (1997) argues that the feminist focus on gender and patriarchy as the source of reproductive repression often overlooks the importance of race and class in shaping our understanding of reproductive liberty and the degree of "choice" that women really have. Similar to technologies that prevent birth, technologies that *assist* birth are also shaped by race and class. Across nations, these new reproductive technologies, despite their "novel" nature, are often more conforming than liberating and tend to reify structures of inequality.

FROM POPULATION CONTROL
TO REPRODUCTIVE TOURISM

How does the use of assisted reproductive technologies like surrogacy fit into this anti-natalist discourse and aggressive population control movement in India? Scholars, within and outside India, have analyzed what they call the "revised eugenics script" in the policies of the (international) population movement (Hartmann 2006). On the one hand, negative eugenics, targeted mainly at minorities, continues with policies like voluntary or incentivized sterilization. On the other hand, positive eugenics has appropriated the language of "individual choices" to strategically emphasize assisted fertility options for upper-class, white couples (Hartmann 2006; Stern 2005). Legal scholar Dorothy Roberts analyzes this "script" in the context of the United States in her book *Killing the Black Body: Race, Reproduction, and the Meaning of Liberty* (1997). Roberts calls it "the proliferation of rhetoric and policies that degrade Black women's procreative decisions" and at the same time reflect the obsession with "creating and preserving genetic ties between white parents and their children" (246). For instance, in the United States in the 1970s, while black Puerto Rican and Indian women were being pressured into this operation, white middle-class women found it nearly impossible to find a doctor who would sterilize them. The "reluctance" of doctors to sterilize white middle-class women continues even today (95). A similar racial disparity can be seen in the access and use of fertility services. For instance, despite the black population having an infertility rate one and half times higher than that of whites, there is a predominant use of ARTs by white couples. This racial disparity is partly based on what Roberts labels "racial steering"—fertility clinics deliberately steering black patients away from ARTs.[7]

Not surprisingly, these current forms of eugenics are complementary to, and often the product of, neoliberal ideologies and policies. For example, the neoliberal concepts of "burden" and "consumer choice" are often used to justify contemporary forms of negative and positive eugenics (Hartmann 2006; Rao 2004). Under neoliberalism, the shrinking of the welfare state can be justified by portraying the poor and people of color as "drains on the economy and the state" and a wasteful burden. Subsequently, negative eugenics, in the form of population control measures and technologies, can target women of color and poor women in the Third World. While the concepts of "waste" and "burden" are intrinsic to negative eugenics, the concept of "consumer choice" is intrinsic to positive eugenics and the promotion of new reproductive technologies (Hartmann 2006).

The revised eugenics script is evident in the policies of the government of India. On the one hand, government expenditure on public health infrastructure is shrinking and poor women are being subjected to population control targets. On the other hand, Indian scientists are investing in new reproductive technologies like test tube babies, IVFs, and surrogacy, and medical tourism (especially in these assisted reproductive services) is booming. Commercial surrogacy is yet another paradox of the post-liberalization era. It is ironic that a country that has the highest absolute number of maternal deaths and only 51 doctors for every 100,000 people is focusing on providing birth-related services to international patients. Reproductive travel and investment in assisted reproductive technologies (ART) continue to flourish, even when infertility constitutes only a small segment of domestic priorities.[8]

But what is the government policy toward Indian women, especially lower-class women, who do indeed require or desire infertility treatment? Here too we see clear indications of eugenics at play. While the Ninth and the Tenth Five-Year Plans committed to ARTs and affiliated services, these services are, in effect, confined to selected tertiary public-sector institutions and the private sector, and therefore they are not accessible for the majority of the population (Qadeer 2010b). Indian social scientist and community health activist Imrana Qadeer astutely summarizes the government's strategy to allow these "red technologies" that are "risky, invasive and unregulated" to flourish in the private sector. This strategy minimizes the risks and costs of primary health care in the public sector and at the same time keeps increasing profits for the private sector (20). As far as the Indian state is concerned, ARTs make good business sense, and whoever can pay for such technologies is actively encouraged to use them.

Unarguably, the history of reproductive politics in India is a story of the state's surveillance and regulation of women's (fertile) bodies. It is also a history of contradictions. When neoliberalism becomes the buzzword, pro-natalist technologies entering an otherwise anti-natalist state lead to explicit instances of what I have called "neo-eugenics." In the next few chapters I demonstrate how the reproductive politics of surrogates in everyday life is in conversation with this form of eugenics. As anthropologist Lawrence Cohen notes about the sterilization operation in India, the narratives of the surrogates reveal not just the "ubiquity of state interventions in their reproductive lives" but also "its intimacy, its identity with or proximity to the everyday" (2005, 87). In essence, on an everyday basis, as surrogates negotiate with the multiple levels of power, in the family and the clinic, their resistive strategies inadvertently speak to the global imperative of lowering the fertility of lower-class women, especially women in the global south.

3   WHEN THE FISH TALK ABOUT THE WATER

FIELD NOTES, 2006, Garv, India: The auto-rickshaw driver looks puzzled when I ask him to take me to the Armaan Maternity Clinic. I would have thought that with the kind of national and international publicity this doctor and her clinic are bringing to the little town of Garv, she would be as famous as any Bollywood movie star. I was right. No one knows the name of the clinic, but everyone knows *the* doctor. "Oh, you want to go to Usha Madam's hospital," the driver replies after realizing what I meant. "Usha Madam is *very* famous. All foreigners go to her. I'll take you there for 10 rupees." So starts my journey through narrow, clustered side streets, full of people on cycles or on foot, competing for space with honking cars, motorcycles, and *thhela waalas* (vendors selling their wares on carts), cows, and stray dogs.

Garv is an uncelebrated Indian city, a strange mix of development and neglect. There are the usual open dustbins, pigs, cows, rotting food, and stinking sewage that are encountered regularly in the smaller cities of India. But in Garv these coexist with high-tech Internet cafés and phone booths offering not just the usual inter-city calling facilities but also international calls and technology like Internet phone service, rarely found even in the capital city of New Delhi. Every second shop sells toilet paper and mineral water (items that are not on the grocery lists of most Indians) and women wearing Benetton T-shirts and tight jeans whiz by on their motorcycles. Amid the rubbish heaps springs a "dollar store," and in a half-finished residential area a "New York" hair salon sits squashed between a dilapidated apartment and a Hindu temple. The signs of modernization in Garv are due in large part to the residents who have settled abroad but regularly return to visit their families. Many end up investing in the local economy and participating in local politics. Locals inform me that with the recent downturn in the economy in the United States, some expatriates have decided to return home for good.

As the auto-rickshaw pulls up outside the Armaan Maternity Clinic, the first thing I notice is how unremarkable it seems—one among the many mushrooming sonography centers, ultrasound clinics, medical stores and clinics lined up one after the other. The big garbage dump right outside the clinic's courtyard is dwarfed by Dr. Usha Khanderia's gleaming luxury car. It's only ten in the morning, but the doctor is doing good business. The place is packed with around 50 women and some men, waiting in lines before me. The women are all dressed in brightly colored synthetic saris. I hear a visibly pregnant woman speaking in English (unusual for this town) on her cell phone. She tells the caller that the baby is doing well and she has come to the clinic for her weekly checkup. I suspect she is someone I will want to talk to later. But for now she will have to wait, as it is time for me to meet the other surrogates.

INITIATION INTO SURROGACY

Clearly, as social scientists we are interpreters, not ventriloquists; we have access to our subjects' mediated representations of themselves and can only portray our own mediated understanding and representation of them as best we can.

—Diane Lauren Wolf, *Factory Daughters*

One could well assume that the contours of the postcolonial anti-natalist state is a given, rarely noticed by the surrogates themselves. As James Scott poetically noted in *Weapons of the Weak* (1985), "One cannot, after all, expect the fish to talk about the water; it is simply the medium in which they live and breathe." But unlike James Scott's Malay peasants who refrained from talking about the "water," the "fish" in this study regularly articulated their interpretation of the state, the clinic, their families, and their role in all these entities. In this chapter I will focus on narratives of recruitment and initiation, which provide an ideal starting point for the exploration of surrogacy as a new form of labor. How many of these women "chose" this occupation, in at least the very literal sense? How many were pushed or coerced into it by brokers and/or family members?

"Choice" is a tricky word, and inarguably all surrogates in this study are financially impoverished. But to validate the choices women make even when they are financially desperate, I identify the women who walked into the clinic on their own accord. Did a surrogate's control over the recruitment process determine her overall experiences of surrogacy? As a scholar of gendered forms of labor, I find the question of choice both intriguing and essential. I confess I made the usual assumptions when first embarking on this research. I assumed that three groups of women—those who *choose* surrogacy, those who are relatively educated, and those who have previously been employed outside of the house—are likely to benefit most from surrogacy and are also likely to have more control over their earnings. But over time, as the complexities of the women's experiences became clear, many of my initial assumptions came undone. The women I interviewed for this study talked at length about their initiation into the surrogacy process. These conversations provided invaluable insight into the surrogates' past, family structure, gender roles, and other demographic patterns relevant to this study. These glimpses into their past shed light on the present: their involvement in surrogacy, their negotiation of different layers of domination, their awareness about the surrogacy processes, and their experiences of surrogacy before the actual delivery.

Once I collected and coded all of the narratives, I observed three types of responses to the recruitment and initiation process. First there were the women who stated that they became surrogates completely of their own accord. This group included women such as Ramya, Dipali, and Parvati. They heard about surrogacy from different sources (often from the media) and came to the clinic without a broker, and sometimes without their husband's permission. In sharp contrast is the second group—women like Yashoda, Regina, Mona, and Sharda—who had no control over the recruitment process. These women were recruited systematically by brokers in the surrogacy trade. The third group comprised women like Rita, Puja, Panna, and Hasomati, who were "convinced" by their in-laws and their husbands. There are some overlaps between the second and third groups, when family members often acted as brokers in the trade and forfeited part of the brokerage fee for their family members.

In the following pages, you will meet some of the women I spoke to during the course of my research. As a feminist ethnographer, it is my intention to highlight the connections between these women's experiences of surrogacy and their education, work experiences, and relationships with their husbands and in-laws, as well as factors more specific to the surrogacy process itself, like method of recruitment into surrogacy and whether they have kept their surrogacy a secret from their community. Their experiences, their stories, illustrate the complex network of factors that ultimately shape the surrogacy experiences of women.

RAMYA, DIPALI, AND PARVATI: "CHOOSING" SURROGACY

"Is there any other occupation left for women in a society as unequal as ours?"

—Ramya, 2006

"There is nothing wrong with surrogacy. I am not hiding this from anyone."

—Dipali, 2007

Name: Ramya
Age: 29
Occupation: Bank teller
Husband's work: Factory worker
Total household income per month: $70
Has delivered a baby girl to a non-resident Indian couple who were settled in the United States

After finishing high school, Ramya worked as a bank teller. It was there that she met a man, fell in love, and got married. Her parents did not want to face the scandal often associated with "love marriages" in India, so Ramya eloped with her boyfriend.[1] For the first ten years of their marriage, Ramya and her husband had a steady income that kept them financially solvent and met their needs and those of their one daughter. Then Ramya's husband lost his job at the bank and had to accept a low-paying job in a factory. Ramya continued to work as a bank teller, but their combined income was not enough to send their daughter to an English-medium (private) school. In 2007, Ramya heard about surrogacy at the Garv clinic on a local news channel, quit her job, and came to the clinic without her husband's permission. When she told her husband, he was furious and insisted that his income was enough for all "reasonable" household expenses. But Ramya wanted to keep sending their daughter to a good school and get her married "in style." She decided to become a surrogate for an Indian couple settled in the United States. Her husband remained reluctant till the end.

Although her in-laws live in the same city, Ramya and her husband live in a separate apartment away from them. Ramya asserts that she chose this living arrangement to prevent her in-laws from "interfering in day-to-day decisions and activities." "I got married twelve years ago, I was very young but I took this decision. I told my husband that I want to live independently. They don't live very far from us. But that way they don't interfere in day-to-day activities and tell me what I can do and cannot do. It's better this way."

Ramya claims that she has a very open relationship with her husband and almost all household decisions, ranging from decisions about contraceptives to the choice of a school for their daughter, are joint decisions.

> My husband and I discuss everything frankly, whether it is about money, taking a loan or the number of children we want to have. I am lucky because we had a love marriage. It's not like with all other couples, we are like friends to each other. We have just one child—a daughter. We had talked about it when I was pregnant the first time and decided irrespective of whether a boy or girl we won't have any more. It's more important to take the best care of just one. So I got an operation (sterilization) done to prevent further pregnancies.[2] But when I read about surrogacy in the newspaper and I realized that I wanted to do this, even if it meant going against his wishes.

Ramya is an exception at many levels. She is one of the most well-educated surrogates, she works in the finance sector, and she self-identifies as a middle-class professional. In almost all her conversations with me she emphasizes that she is very different from the rest of the surrogates—perhaps as an attempt to negotiate the stigma attached to women who sell their wombs out of sheer financial desperation.

> I used to work in the finance sector, and my husband is a professional as well. It's just that our situation has become very bad lately. That's why I have to do this. You know I am a Brahman [upper caste] and everyone else in my family is very well off—some are in the U.S., some are rich businessmen. If they wanted they could get us "set" in just one day. But we don't want to ask them. I'd rather do this than beg for money from relatives.

Ramya plans to use the money to pay for her daughter's education and dowry. She is the only surrogate who was initially reluctant to discuss her surrogacy experience with me. She constantly worries that the stigma of surrogacy will pass on to her daughter, and she refuses to reveal her true identity, even to women who share the clinic room with her.

> If this were a big city like Mumbai or Delhi it would have been different. But in Garv people are very narrow-minded. They don't understand the science of this process—the fact that the eggs and the sperms are mixed in the lab. They think it's like a normal baby so I must be having a relationship [sex] with the man [intended father]. If I had a son I wouldn't worry about what people say. But I have a daughter and I don't want the stigma of surrogacy to affect her chances of getting married later on.

Although Ramya claims that she has a very open and loving relationship with her husband, other surrogates remarked that he has never visited her at the hostel. The doctor encourages surrogates to live in dormitory-style hostels. In 2013 there were three such hostels, financed and managed by the clinic. A matron appointed by the doctor monitors the diet, health, and even the leisure-time activities of the surrogates living in this hostel. (I discuss the disciplinary regime and the "making of a perfect surrogate" in these hostels in chapter 4.) Ramya admits that her husband came to the clinic just to sign the consent form and has not visited her even once in the three months that she has been at the hostel. Ramya has not revealed her pregnancy to anyone in her family, community, or village. She recognizes that the secrecy surrounding surrogacy and the subsequent isolation at the clinic and hostel make the surrogacy experience more painful.

◆ ◆ ◆

But not all surrogates keep their surrogacy a secret. Like Ramya, surrogate Dipali chose to become a surrogate without consulting anyone in her family. But unlike Ramya, Dipali made her decision known to everyone in her family.

Name: Dipali
Age: 25
Occupation: Insurance agent
Separated from husband
Total household income per month: $30
Surrogate for an Indian couple settled in South Africa

Dipali is one of the few surrogates to have completed her high school education. She wanted to get an undergraduate degree in commerce, but her father, a clerk in a government office and father of four, could not afford to send her to college. He got her married instead. Dipali had her first child at the age of 17, less than a year after marriage. When her second child was barely six months old, Dipali ran away from her abusive husband and took refuge at her brother's house in a city close to Mumbai. Dipali says, "I can do anything for children. My children are the main reason why I moved away from him [her husband]. He used to hit me, get angry in front of them. I had to leave. . . . See nowadays a woman can never be sure whether her marriage will last. You can't kill yourself if it doesn't nor can you sacrifice your children's future."

Dipali read about surrogacy in a newspaper in 2006 and started looking for surrogacy options all over India. She tried to be a surrogate in a fertility clinic in Mumbai, but the clinic did not take surrogacy cases, so she came to Garv instead. After donating her eggs three times, she started the treatment to become a surrogate mother. Dipali is also a self-proclaimed broker and brings other women—mostly her colleagues from work—to be egg donors at the clinic. She wants to use the money to stay independent and not be a "burden" on her brother anymore.

> I get a very small commission, Rs 200 [$5] for the egg donors I bring to the clinic. I want to make my own flat with the money I get out of this surrogacy. I don't want to be dependent on anyone—neither my parents nor my brothers. I know I should go back to work in the insurance company but I don't think that's the best option for me. My children are getting older and they will need someone to help them with homework. Who will do all that if I am at work? That's why I've decided I'll do this again.

Dipali decided not to keep her surrogacy a secret. Once she was accepted by the clinic, she managed to get the consent of her entire family. She has not only informed them about her decision to become a surrogate, but she also has their support and involvement. Although she faced a lot of resistance and disapproval in the beginning, by her third trimester she had all of them by her side: "There is nothing wrong with surrogacy. I am not hiding this from anyone. I brought my entire family—my parents and my elder brother, who has studied medicine—to meet Dr. Khanderia. And now that all of them have agreed, I have no tension. My mother will [take] care of my children when I am here. She supports me in everything. After the delivery I'll go back to my house, take good food, rests and medicine and come back for the second time."

◆ ◆ ◆

Like Dipali, Parvati actively chose to become a surrogate and decided not to keep her surrogacy a secret from her family.

Name: Parvati
Age: 36
Occupation: Nurse
Husband's work: Factory worker
Total household income per month: $100
Hired as a surrogate by clients from Mumbai, India

Parvati got married at 17. When I met her in 2006, she was 36 and had a 15-year-old son. She had been working as a nurse in a hospital but left the job when she got into surrogacy. Although she calls herself a nurse, Parvati admits that she failed her middle school exams and never went back to school again. She loves to read but hates mathematics and the sciences. She always wanted to be a teacher but was not educated enough to become one. Her usual tasks at the hospital are cleaning the equipment, making sure the room is clean and the bedpan and linen are changed regularly. A doctor at the hospital told her about surrogacy and egg donation.

When I came here the first time the doctor said I was too old to donate eggs but I could try for surrogacy. This was in 2004. There was a couple from New Zealand and they agreed to pay rupees two lakhs [$5,000]. But my husband heard bad things about surrogacy from some of his friends and he didn't let me go ahead with it. After six months we thought if others are doing it why not us. We need the money desperately. . . . We have [a] farm in the village but the land is not fertile and then there is the rising expense of sending our boy to school. We have no savings. We have been staying in a rented house for ten years; the rent, the electricity, and our daily expenses eat away all the earnings.

Parvati and her husband live in a village about 20 kilometers from her in-laws. Her in-laws are old and ailing, and Parvati has to spend part of her income and much of her time looking after them.

> We moved away from them because of my husband's work. I sometimes feel we made a mistake. It is a bigger problem for me to travel every day to go see them. Also I got no help in raising my son—I had to manage single-handedly, with no help of elders. It was even more difficult because I don't sit at home—I've been working as a nurse for over 10 years now. But other surrogates here tell me I am lucky to be staying away from my in-laws. They wouldn't have allowed me to become a surrogate at this age.

Parvati has been at the hostel for more than two months, but her husband, a worker in a food-processing factory, rarely visits her. Parvati does not complain. She says he is a very good husband, although she admits that he is too "clumsy" to do any housework.

> My husband is very good, he consults me for most big expenses. Otherwise you know how it is in most homes—the man keeps all his income and also takes away the woman's earnings. It's not like that at our home. He gives me some of his money for household expenses. All my money goes towards my son's education. He [her husband] doesn't really know anything about housework. He is very clumsy and cannot even take a glass of water by himself! But you can't really expect men to be able to deal with the kitchen. I'm used to it, I've been managing alone for such a long time now—since we moved away from my in-laws. My son helps me out with the bigger chores. Of course, nowadays I have a maid who does all the housework.

Parvati hopes to use the money to build a house and save on the monthly rent. Although the money is not enough to build a real house, she is hoping the intended parents would pay some extra money because she is carrying twins. She is one of the few to have not kept the surrogacy a secret from her family and community. I never heard Parvati complain about any aspect of her surrogacy experience, partly because she had the support of her entire family. Unlike Ramya and most other surrogates who decide to keep their surrogacy a secret from their community and consequently have little family support, Parvati had different visitors during lunch hour every day. But like many other husbands, her husband is conspicuously missing from these family visits. Parvati's succinct explanation for her husband's behavior: "If he can't do it [have sex], why would he bother visiting me?"

◆ ◆ ◆

While women like Dipali, Ramya, and Parvati are active decision makers from the very beginning of their surrogacy experience, there are others who are pushed into surrogacy by brokers. Unlike the first set of women, the second group—Regina, Yashoda, Sharda, and Mona—did not read about surrogacy in the papers. All four were initially very reluctant to get involved in such a stigmatized occupation, but they were systematically recruited by brokers in the trade.

REGINA, YASHODA, SHARDA, AND MONA: BROKERED INTO SURROGACY

"It sounded so wrong. But she [the broker] knows my situation and was able to convince me."

—Regina, 2006

"How can a widow get pregnant, that too with some stranger's baby? I did not want to do this but Vimla [the broker] convinced me."

—Yashoda, 2007

Name: Regina
Age: 45
Occupation: Maid
Husband's occupation: Rickshaw puller
Total household income per month: $30
Surrogate for an Indian couple settled in Dubai

Regina's marriage was arranged by her parents, against her wishes, at the age of 16. She moved in with her 90-year-old father-in-law and a husband twice her age in a village more than 100 miles away from her parents. Her husband turned out to be neither as rich as was promised by his parents nor as loving. After the death of her father-in-law, Regina decided to take up a job as a maid. She works in seven different houses, cleaning and washing for more than 12 hours a day.

Vimla, a nurse and a broker in the trade, brought Regina to the clinic. Vimla had a hard time convincing her even though Regina needed the money desperately. Regina has a daughter with severe mental challenges, a son who needs to be sent to school, and a husband who is a "useless alcoholic."

> I just wasn't sure I wanted to do this thing. It sounded so wrong. But she [Vimla] knows my situation and was able to convince me. Of course I had to pay a lot of money to her as brokerage fee. She knows my husband is a rickshaw puller and earns according to the day. It's not our rickshaw so he has to pay the owner half of what he earns per day and there is hardly anything left over at the end of the day. He brings back only Rs 25 per day [50 cents]. On top of that, he is a useless alcoholic. I work as a maid in many people's houses and earn about Rs 500 per month [$10]. We have a little room of our own but this money is not enough for anything.

Regina runs the household single-handedly and makes almost all of the household decisions independent of her husband. She decided not to keep her surrogacy a secret from anyone in her family or community: "I've told everyone I am doing this. What's the point in hiding this—they'll come to know in any case. I can't possibly tell them that I am having my own baby at the age of 45. But I am not telling anyone how much I'm going to make from this surrogacy, not even my husband, *especially* not my husband. He is a useless alcoholic and I don't want him to know about the money."

◆ ◆ ◆

Like Regina, Yashoda is one of the few surrogates to take all decisions independent of her husband and in-laws. But while Regina talks about her independence and decisions with incredible confidence and élan, Yashoda is hesitant and apprehensive.

Name: Yashoda
Age: 38
Occupation: Maid in a clinic
Widow
Total household income per month: $25
Surrogate for a single man from Spain

Yashoda's husband died 12 years ago when her son was barely a year old. She has been working as a maid in a hospital to send her daughter to college and her son to school, but it has been very hard, both emotionally and financially. She has a mud house, but it legally belongs to her mother-in-law. Yashoda faces constant harassment from her mother-in-law but is forced to live with them. Her monthly income as a maid is never going to be enough to buy her another hut.

Yashoda read about surrogacy in a newspaper but was too scared to mention it to her in-laws. In 2007, Vimla came to Yashoda's village in search of eligible women, heard about "Yashoda the widow," and knocked on her door. Yashoda recalls:

> I read about surrogacy in a paper but I was reluctant to come to Garv. How can a widow get pregnant, that too with some stranger's baby? What would people say? [She starts crying.] I did not want to do this but broker Vimla convinced me that the kind of struggle I have to go through just to survive is not worth it. She is the one who eventually got me here. I had to pay Rs 10,000 to her as brokerage fee [$200]. My mother-in-law looks after my children while I am here. I knew she would harass me even more so I didn't tell her why I am in Garv. I've lied to her and said I've got a job as a nanny.

Although Yashoda has kept her surrogacy a secret from her in-laws, her children are not only aware of their mother's decision but are also supportive. They visit her every day and bring tea and snacks for her. Yashoda wants to use the money to rent an apartment or build a hut away from her in-laws. She would save the rest for her son's higher education.

> This is the first time that I am not giving up all my income to my mother-in-law. Whatever I earned as a maid I had to surrender to her and she would decide how much spending money my children and I would get every month. This is the first time I get to keep all of it with me. I get to decide what I want to do with it. I know this money is not enough for everything. I know I will go back to being a maid. But as long as it gets me out of that house—I think all this will be worth it.

◆ ◆ ◆

Like Yashoda and Regina, Sharda was recruited into surrogacy by a broker connected to Armaan clinic.

Name: Sharda
Age: 38
Occupation: Housewife
Husband's work: Works in a printing plant
Total household income per month: $40
Hired as a surrogate by clients from Maharashtra, India

Sharda and her husband are from the same village. They went to the same school, but both left during middle school. Sharda has been married for 21 years and had her first child at the age of 20.

> Both of us are equally educated—or equally uneducated, you can say! But he is much smarter that I am about everyday things. He has a good position in the printing press. It's just that the press is doing badly so they can't pay him well enough. He wanted me to work as well, but I never really got any job. He didn't want me to work as a maid in anyone's house— that is one of the only things I could have done with my education.

Sharda's neighbor, a nurse at the clinic, told her about surrogacy and got her to the clinic. Her husband accompanied her on her first visit.

> What do I understand of surrogacy? I just know that it's his [the intended father's] sperm that is put in me and from that a son is born. I need regular injections and medicines for that. When I came here they made me do some paperwork. It said that I know what I am doing and we take full responsibility. They asked my husband to sign as well. My husband understands all this much better. I think he read the whole contract and all the papers.

Sharda's husband seems to be the one keeping track of all the payments received. But Sharda seems to be more aware than she admits: "You should ask him how much we have got till now. [She asks her husband.] Rs two lakhs [$4,000]? [Her husband nods.] He has decided what to do with the money—educate our children. My daughter has her exams coming up—English exam. And also build our own house—we live in a rented house."

Although Sharda claims that her husband makes all the decisions and does all the "money talk," I often hear her advising him on money matters and even rebuking him on certain decisions. During one of his visits she explains to him, "This is not social service we are doing. We need the money. I want to be able to put something away in the bank for later. So go remind her [the matron] that they [the intended parents] still haven't paid the full second installment. You can't postpone it anymore."

Sharda and her husband seem to have an unusually equitable division of household chores. While Sharda is in the clinic, her husband takes care of all the housework. She explains: "My parents and my mother-in-law passed away a long time ago. There are no other women in the family who can help him. But he knows how to do everything except make *roti* [bread]. Even when I am at home he cleans up after himself and even washes the children's clothes."

Although Sharda's husband is the one ostensibly handling the finances, Sharda is aware of both the process involved in surrogacy and the payments involved. Perhaps because there are no other options, Sharda's husband single-handedly manages child care and household chores while Sharda is at the clinic. It is worth noting that in most other cases, female kin take up these responsibilities; it is unusual for the husband to be so involved. (I discuss changes in the gendered division of labor within the surrogate's family in the epilogue.)

◆ ◆ ◆

The story of the next surrogate—Mona—has many parallels with Sharda's life story. Mona believes that her husband is the one in control of the surrogacy payments and makes all related decisions. But in practice, Mona seems to have a surprisingly equitable relationship with her husband and is much more aware of the process and payments than she admits.

Name: Mona
Age: 24
Occupation: Housewife; used to work in a pharmacy
Husband's work: Factory worker
Total household income per month: $70
Hired by Indian clients settled in the United States

Mona grew up in Nepal in a middle-class household. Her father was an engineer with a government department and sent both his daughters to a good school. Mona has completed high school, and her father was willing to send her to college as well, but Mona was not interested in studying any further. At age 17 she got married and moved to India with her husband when he got a job in a small plastics factory. Mona used to work in a pharmacy, earning almost as much as her husband does at the factory, but she left her work once both her children started going to school.

Mona heard about surrogacy from one of her neighbors—a surrogacy broker. She charged Mona Rs 10,000 ($200) for bringing her to the clinic. Mona recalls her first day at the clinic:

> I was so scared that I was shivering. She [the neighbor] took care of everything—from hearing what the doctor had to say, following all the names of medicines, understanding what injection has to be given to me and when. I was just nodding away at whatever they said. My husband was not happy with this but I convinced him to come for the next session. He understands the payment system and will meet the couple. I did not pay attention to anything. He took the money and he must have kept it in the bank. I don't know.

Mona is staying in a surrogacy hostel and will continue to stay there till her delivery. But she says she is not worried about her children, a six-year-old daughter and a four-year-old son. Her husband would take care of them.

> He knows how to do everything. He used to help me even before I started this, especially on Sundays. During my pregnancy [when she was pregnant with her first child] I used to work in the day shift. He would take care of the house and at night he would go for work. I guess that's why he is not having any trouble taking care of the house now. He has stopped going for work now since he has to take care of the children.

Mona's husband seems to be an exceptional case in terms of his involvement in household chores. Mona explains, "Actually when I got married I didn't know anything. He taught me how to manage all the household chores. I was pampered a lot when I stayed with my parents. We were quite well off and my parents wanted me to study. I guess that's why he knows how to take care of everything."

Mona and her husband will use the money to build a small house and save the rest for their children's education and marriage. Although Mona says she lets her husband deal with the finances and make all the decisions about how the money should be spent, she seems to have a fair idea about the monthly payments and installments as well as how she would want the money to be spent: "The couple said they will pay us 2.5 lakhs [$5,000] and Rs. 2,000 per month [$40]. The monthly payments they make pays for this hostel and the rest keeps our household running. I'll get the second installment when I complete the next three months. I suggested to my husband that we should use the first installment to buy a piece of land."

◆ ◆ ◆

While Yashoda, Regina, Mona, and Sharda have all been brought into surrogacy by brokers, their experiences of surrogacy are disparate. Despite her initial apprehensions about surrogacy and her apparent meek nature, Yashoda manages to retain control over the earnings partly because she has no husband to negotiate with—she is a widow. Regina shares Yashoda's broker but not her meek personality. She manages to keep her husband out of the surrogacy arrangement and is confident that she will control the entire earnings. Finally in this recruitment category are two other women—Mona and Sharda. Both claim that their husbands manage the finances, but in practice, both are aware not only of the process but also the payments involved. Mona and Sharda seem to be overcompensating for their role as temporary breadwinners by downplaying their awareness.

The final category of surrogates includes women who are "convinced" by their in-laws and husbands. Although commercial brokers are assumed to be the most exploitative aspect of the recruitment process, instances of manipulation by family members can be just as exploitative, if not more so. Once again, it is vital to pay attention to the disparate experiences of the women within this category—the initiation does not determine their ultimate experience of surrogacy.

PANNA, HASOMATI, SUDHA, PUJA, AND RITA: SURRENDERING TO FAMILY?

"I don't know if the egg is mine or not. I wasn't involved in the paperwork either."

—Panna, 2007

"I was so scared. I didn't want to do all this. But my husband agreed, so I had to come with them to the clinic."

—Hasomati, 2007

Name: Panna
Age: 27
Occupation: Housewife
Husband's work: Sells bangles in a cart
Total household income per month: $60
Hired as a surrogate by clients from Turkey

Panna spent her childhood helping her parents on their farm and has never been to school. She got married at the age of 19 and is the mother of three children. Though she never went to a formal school, Panna has a great desire for learning, especially embroidery and other crafts. She wanted to start a small sewing business from the house, but her father-in-law prohibited her. Now, after her father-in-law's death, she wants to get her husband's permission and start the business. For now, however, they have barely enough money to pay the monthly bills, and Panna does not want to think of investing in her business. Despite their financial desperation, Panna did not want to become a surrogate. Her sister-in-law persuaded her to go to the clinic and meet the doctor. Panna talks about her first day at the clinic:

> I don't know where my husband and my sister-in-law heard about this [surrogacy] but once they had the idea of making me a surrogate, they just would not give up. When I refused, my husband came to [the] clinic and met up with Doctor Madam instead. He came home and told me about other women at the clinic, and told me it looked safe. But even when they [her sister-in-law and her husband] were putting me in the auto-rickshaw and I was on my way to the clinic, I was crying.

I meet Panna four months after the embryo transfer when she is well into the second trimester of her pregnancy. But she seems to have very little idea of about the surrogacy process.

> When I came here the first time Doctor Madam explained to me what surrogacy is but I didn't really understand. My sister-in-law told me a few things as well, you know, about how the baby will be made. [She giggles.]

I don't know if the egg is mine or not. I wasn't involved in the paperwork either. When the nurse was explaining everything to us, my husband was there. He understands more about all this and he is the one who is handling the money. You should talk to him, or my sister-in-law.

Panna introduces me to her sister-in-law, who tells me that the intended parents used donor eggs and agreed to pay $4,000. Her sister-in-law seems to be managing the finances of the family. She tells me that they want to spend the money to pay back some debt and start a small family business in garments. Panna does not seem to be aware of these plans.

Panna lives with her in-laws, who visit her regularly at the clinic, but she decided not to tell her parents: "I decided not to tell them. I know they would not have approved of their daughter doing such a thing. There is no point telling them, they couldn't have done anything to stop this. My husband is taking care of everything. I am not worried."

◆ ◆ ◆

Like Panna, Hasomati seems to have very little idea about the surrogacy contract. She also was brought to the clinic by the combined efforts of her husband and her sister-in-law and leaves the financial transaction to her college-educated husband.

Name: Hasomati
Age: 31
Occupation: Works at home
Husband's work: Works in a garment factory
Total household income per month: $40
Hired as a surrogate by Indian clients settled in Dubai

Hasomati has been married for 15 years and had her first child when she was barely 15. She has never been to high school, but her husband is college-educated. Her ambition is to send both her sons to an English-medium school. She lives with her in-laws in a big city, 40 miles away from Garv. Her sister-in-law lives in Garv and heard about surrogacy from her neighbor, a nurse at the clinic.

My sister knew about our desperate condition. So when she heard about surrogacy at this clinic she came home and tried to convince me to try it. She told me, "You have no earnings, your house needs to be built, and your boy is going to enter high school. He'll probably need tuitions for his exams. Why don't you at least come with me to the Garv clinic?" I was so scared. I didn't want to do all this. But my husband agreed, so I had to come with them to the clinic.

Hasomati is in her second trimester but has little knowledge of the surrogacy process. Although Divya, the counselor at the clinic, is expected to explain the entire process to the surrogates and mediate meetings between the clients and the surrogates, Hasomati says she had no such meeting or counseling: "My party [couple hiring her] is from Dubai but I haven't really spoken to them. Maybe my husband has, I don't know about that. I am not sure what the contract says since my husband read and signed the contract. I only passed middle school but he went to college. He understands these things more. No, Divya *didi* [elder sister] hasn't explained anything to me. Well, I am illiterate, I guess that's why?"

Hasomati's husband visits her every weekend. Her sister-in-law usually accompanies him. They advised Hasomati not to tell her parents, in case they demanded a share in the payment. Hasomati agrees with their decision: "My husband is a busy man, he can't take care of the house. I've told my in-laws I am doing this and they help with the household chores, sending the children to school and everything. Why tell my parents and cause more heartache to them? They will not be happy to hear that I am doing this. I don't think they would want any money; they have a farm of their own. But they will be unhappy."

◆ ◆ ◆

Sudha's initiation into surrogacy was very similar to that of Hasomati and Panna. Sudha's sister-in-law, a surrogacy broker, brought her to the clinic.

Name: Sudha
Age: 27
Occupation: Works on a farm
Husband's work: Truck driver

Total household income per month: $30
Hired by clients from Mumbai, India

Sudha was raised in a village where both her parents were contract workers on someone else's farm. They never had enough to eat and were
always in debt. Sudha and her brothers have never been to school. At the
age of 14 Sudha got married to a man double her age, from a landowning
family a few miles away from her village. She moved in with her husband
and her in-laws but soon realized that the land they owned was mostly
barren and worth nothing. Sudha and her husband moved to the city in
search of work, and her husband became a truck driver. He comes back
home only once every fortnight. Her in-laws live in a village two hours
away from them.

Sudha heard about surrogacy from her sister-in-law, Vimla, one of the
brokers at the Garv clinic. She offered Sudha a discounted brokerage fee
of $100 for arranging the deal. When her husband is away, Sudha's sister-
in-law is her only kin in the city and Sudha could not refuse.

> What could I have done? She is the only one I know in the city and when
> she asked me to do this, I had to agree. I know we need the money but I
> really didn't want to do this. We survive with what he [her husband] earns,
> why get into something like this? When my husband heard what Vimla
> didi had done, he was very angry at first. But she convinced him that it's
> all for our good and maybe with the money we earn he can buy an auto-
> rickshaw of his own.

Even in her seventh month of pregnancy, Sudha is very bitter about her
situation. Her husband has quit his truck driving job and is taking care of
the finances. He visits her once a week and brings their son with him. The
doctor has allowed Sudha's daughter to stay with Sudha at the clinic—an
exception made by the doctor because Sudha has no kin in the city who
can take care of the girl in her absence. Their monthly expenses ($50) are
paid for by the couple hiring Sudha. Sudha has not seen a single rupee of
the money she has earned.

> I want to build a house in the village and I want to send our children to
> school. Many of their friends go to school and I know they would be very
> good students. But ever since Vimla didi has given him this idea, he only
> wants to buy an auto-rickshaw. Even for the contract signing, they took

only my husband's signature. He knows everything. I haven't seen even one rupee of the payment. I know the child inside me is not mine, but I am happy that it will be luckier than my own children.

◆ ◆ ◆

Sudha's, Hasomati's, and Panna's experiences of surrogacy are a clear indication of the exploitative potential of surrogacy arrangements for women. More than half of the women I interviewed heard about surrogacy from formal and informal brokers, and many of the rest were urged or coerced to become surrogates by their family members. These women have very little awareness of the medical processes involved in surrogacy and often have no control over the payment, either. Their bodies are subjected to weeks of injections, treatment, and surveillance without their awareness and consent. It would be incorrect, however, to deduce that the recruitment structure determines experiences of surrogacy. There are others, like Puja and Rita, who are pushed into surrogacy by their family but manage to regain control over the process and payment.

Name: Puja

Age: 27

Occupation: Worked in a store

Husband's occupation: House painter

Total household income per month: $50

Delivered a baby boy for an Indian couple (2006), underwent hormonal treatment to become a surrogate for an Indian couple settled in the United States but had a miscarriage (2007), delivered a baby boy to a couple from Canada (2009), surrogate for clients from Delhi (2011)

Puja was born in a village near Garv. She loved going to school and regrets having studied only until the beginning of middle school. But her father, a postman and the sole breadwinner for a family of seven, decided to send her three brothers to school instead. Puja wants a better life for her children: "You know I had always dreamt of being an air hostess. But when I saw the situation at home—with my father earning so little—I knew I couldn't study anymore. Both my husband and I haven't had much schooling but I don't want my children to have the same fate. All our income goes in just rent and food. What if my daughter wants to go for higher education—wants to be a doctor or an engineer—where will I get the money to educate her?"

Puja was brought to the clinic by her sister-in-law, a nurse and an informal broker. For this service she charged a percentage of the first installment. Puja admits that she agreed without knowing anything about the process: "I agreed to come to the clinic because I am scared of my sister-in-law. I agreed to do this without knowing much about it. At the clinic the nurse told me that there is nothing immoral about surrogacy. But even when I was getting the seed [embryo] transferred I had no idea what was going on."

Although Puja was pushed into surrogacy by her sister-in-law, she managed to have control over the payments received, buy a plot of land, and keep some money aside in a bank for her children. In 2007 she decided to become a surrogate again despite objections by her father-in-law: "People ask me why I am doing this [surrogacy] again. I know I could have joined the store I used to work in earlier. But there you have to work for at least 12 hours a day and I can't really join work until I have regained strength from my earlier delivery. I told everyone in my family that I am doing this. My father-in-law was very against it. But I told him it's my life, I'll do what I feel is right."

◆ ◆ ◆

Rita's story aligns with that of Puja. Rita was a member of one of the first families to get into the "business of surrogacy." Their mother, an informal broker in the trade, nudged Rita and her sisters into surrogacy.

Name: Rita

Age: 29

Occupation: Housewife

Husband's work: Collects plastic (bottles, etc.) from the street and trash cans

Total household income per month: $40

Has delivered a baby girl for an Indian couple settled in the United States (2006), delivered another baby for another Indian client settled in the United States (2007), and was pregnant with twins for clients from Australia (2011)

Rita got married at the age of 18 and moved in with her husband and her in-laws in a village close to Garv. She had her first child (a girl) one year after marriage and a son a few years later. She lives with her husband in a hut that belonged to her (recently deceased) in-laws. She confesses that her relationship with her "witch-like" mother-in-law was always less than cordial.

> Thankfully, in just three years of our getting married both my in-laws died, first my mother-in-law and then my father-in-law. No, it's not that all mother-in-laws are like witches, but mine was and so is my sister's mother-in-law, a total witch. But I am not mild-mannered like my sister, tolerating all kind of nonsense from her mother-in-law. My mother-in-law tried to harass me once and I beat her up! She wanted full control over our money, my kitchen, and my children and then she tried to hit me when I argued back. What could I have done? I had to hit her back. If she had killed me what would have happened to my children? She stopped misbehaving with me after the beating I gave her. Now they are both dead. (She laughs.) No, I didn't kill them! But now there is no one to bother me. If they had been alive, they would not have allowed me to become a surrogate.

Rita's story, especially her aggressive retaliation to the harassment by her in-laws, is not a usual one. But the conclusion is just the strongest version of what I heard from many other surrogates—the presence of in-laws shapes the surrogacy experiences of women. In-laws often forbid their daughter-in-law from becoming a surrogate, or if they do allow it, they often control the earnings.

Rita was urged by her mother, Kanta, a nurse and broker at the clinic, to start by donating eggs at the clinic and then to become a surrogate. Rita's husband, Alok, was very reluctant at the beginning, but her mother persuaded him to give his consent. Rita talks about her decision to become a surrogate for the second time in two years:

> They [the intended parents] liked me so much they came back for me. The first time they paid Rs. 2 lakhs [$4,000] for it. This time they have raised the pay by Rs. 25,000 [$500]. I know maybe one time was enough and I shouldn't be greedy but what do I do? I really want to educate my daughter. She loves to go to school. In her school when they ask her what she wants to be when she grows up, she says "I want to be like

Doctor Madam." . . . I am not very educated. I wanted to go to college but couldn't because of our financial situation. If I had been better educated I wouldn't have had to do this. I don't want my daughter to be in such a desperate situation.

Rita used the money from her first surrogacy to make household repairs. She wants to use the payment from her second surrogacy to send her daughter to college. Although she says that she and her husband decide on household expenditures jointly, in all her conversations, she talks about "her" money and how "she" wants to spend it. Rita's fiery nature is revealed in almost all moments of her life story—her ability to fight back against her in-laws, to persuade her husband to allow her to become a surrogate, and to have control over the money earned through surrogacy.

Although Rita is not an exception, her relationship with her husband does appear to be unusually equitable. Unlike most other husbands, Alok visits his wife every day, and often brings the children with him. He gives Rita regular updates on the children's homework and seems to be comfortable in his (albeit temporary) role as the primary caregiver. Rita calls Alok a "useful and good" husband:

My husband really takes care of me nowadays. Sometimes he feeds me with his own hands. During the delivery [of her first surrogate child] he was very nervous and would almost cry. He was worried that if something happens to me everyone would criticize him for letting his wife do such a risky thing. He is not useless like all other men. He takes care of the children while I am here [in the surrogacy hostel]. He helped out a little bit with the children earlier as well. He is a good husband, with money, with his habits, everything. He doesn't drink and he doesn't spend excessively. Our household expenses are decided by both of us, there is no one who is the boss, I would say.

Beyond the initial push and shove by family members, surrogacy seems to be a very well-thought-out decision for both Puja and Rita. Puja knows how she wants to spend the money and has decided to become a second-time surrogate despite objections by her father-in-law. Rita, another second-time surrogate, makes all her decisions "jointly" with her husband and has devised a strategy to better their lives with the money earned through surrogacy.

SURROGACY EXPERIENCES: INITIATION, INDEPENDENCE, AND ISOLATION

Whether nudged into surrogacy by their family, nurses, or brokers, or of their own accord, all the women I met at the Garv clinic were motivated by the sheer need for money. Some, like Dipali and Yashoda, became surrogates as a way to get out of abusive relationships and live independently with their children. Many hoped to spend the money on building a hut of their own or starting a small business for their husbands. Others regretted their lack of education and expressed the desire to send their daughters to college. While the need for money binds all of these women together, their experiences of surrogacy are vastly disparate. What is it that shapes the women's experience of surrogacy?

Given the sample size and data I gathered, I hesitate to make any grand connections between a woman's demographic profile and her level of control over the contract negotiations and the money she earned as a surrogate. There were some clear trends, though. For example, living with in-laws increased the chances that the in-laws would stake claims on the earnings. This was more pronounced in cases like Hasomati's and Panna's, where the in-laws were the ones who persuaded the women to become surrogates in the first place. But co-residence with in-laws did not translate into reduced control for one surrogate—Puja. Puja appears to be the primary decision maker, and even defies the authority of her in-laws to become a surrogate. The presence of in-laws was not always detrimental for the surrogates. There were other women, like Hasomati, who had been pushed into surrogacy by their in-laws and had little knowledge about the contract, but also got the constant support and company of their family. It would be simplistic to assert that such women were necessarily worse off than so-called independent women like Ramya, who spent the nine months of surrogacy in total isolation.

Another trend that emerged from my fieldwork was the connection between women who worked outside the house and the degree of control they asserted over the surrogacy process. Ramya, Puja, Regina, and Dipali, who are among those who work outside the house, were more involved with the surrogacy contract than those who have never worked outside the house. Second-time surrogates, like Rita and Puja, also seem to be not just more aware but also much more confident of their decision and in control of their experiences and the payments. I discuss this in more detail in the epilogue, where I revisit many of the surrogates after delivery of the babies.

Women with relatively equitable relationships with their husbands, and those who made household decisions jointly with their husbands, in general did have more say and control over the surrogacy decisions as well. But some surrogates, like Puja and Sharda, treated the incomes earned from surrogacy as special, earnings that they could rightfully control. It is important to point out that the concept of "control over earnings" itself needs to be unpacked. While there were some extremes in which the surrogates either had obvious "control" over the income earned or none at all, there were other situations that fell in the middle. Some of the women, like Sharda and Mona, claimed that their husbands managed the finances. But in practice, both were aware not only of the process but also of the payments involved. These women could be overcompensating for their role as temporary breadwinners but may well be strategically taking this decision.

Education of the surrogate did not have any obvious effect on the level of awareness and involvement with the contract. Divya and Ramya, with college education and active understanding of the contract, can be treated as outliers. In most other cases, education did not determine control and awareness. There were women like Rita and Regina, with hardly any education, who were well versed in the details of the payment and contract. Education did, however, affect women's understanding of the medical processes involved. Again, of all my respondents only Divya and Ramya had knowledge and understanding of all the processes involved in gestational surrogacy. This mystification about the many processes involved was, in part, a conscious strategy of the clinic. I discuss in chapters 4 and 5 how this process of mystification is inherent in the disciplinary strategy of the clinic and has intriguing effects on the everyday negotiations of surrogacy by the women.

The complexities of the women's experiences challenged my main hypothesis—that recruitment structure shapes women's experience of surrogacy. Thus, despite the presence of brokers, women like Puja and Regina are able to have control over their surrogacy experiences and payment received. In fact, women who were "pushed" into surrogacy by formal brokers were more likely to make autonomous decisions beyond the recruitment stage than women who were "convinced" by their family members. In the latter case, the family members (in-laws and husbands) continued to control the finances.

Although my main focus in this chapter has been on women's control over their earnings, the level of family support critically affected women's experiences of surrogacy at the clinic and hostel, and this in turn fundamentally shaped my own understanding of women's experience of surrogacy in Armaan. Many surrogates kept their surrogacy a secret from their families. Exceptions were surrogates like Dipali, Parvati, Puja, and Rita, who openly discussed their decision to become a surrogate with their families. For these women, surrogacy was not an immoral act to be done clandestinely. Subsequently, their days in the clinic were spent not in isolation but in the company of and with the support of their family members. Then there were others, like Ramya, who actively chose to become surrogates, were aware and in control of the money, but detested the process and the isolation. The limited familial support and isolation at the clinic led women to forge alternative kin ties instead. I explore these creative and often powerful connection in chapter 8.

Recruitment, however, is just one step in the whole process of surrogacy. In chapter 4 I analyze the other steps involved in the making of the surrogate and demonstrate that the perfect commercial surrogate is not found ready-made, waiting to be recruited. The perfect surrogate is actively *produced* in fertility clinics and surrogacy hostels.

4 ❧ MANUFACTURING THE PERFECT
MOTHER-WORKER

*Everything works like clockwork. We wake up at 8 am, have tea, take our medicines
and injections and go back to sleep. Then we wake up at noon, bathe and eat lunch.
We basically rest. That's what is required of us. We are allowed visitors but not for the
night. In the evening we pray. Then the English tutor comes and teaches us how to
speak in English. We will be learning how to use a computer next.*

—Tina, a surrogate mother, describing the timetable
at a surrogacy hostel in Garv, 2007

FEMINIST ETHNOGRAPHERS have often ventured to factories and global assembly lines to watch gender at work on the shop floor. Their research demonstrated that good labor—cheap, docile, and dexterous—is not found ready-made. It is produced in the "meaningful practices and rhetorics of shop-floor life" (Salzinger 1993, 16). Like the perfect laborer of global production, a perfect commercial surrogate is not found ready-made in India. The perfect surrogate—"cheap, docile, selfless and nurturing"—is produced in the fertility clinics and surrogacy hostels.

But the story of the production of the perfect surrogate worker is complicated by the fact that the surrogate is required to view herself as both a worker-producer and a mother-reproducer. The disciplinary project devised by the commercial surrogacy regime exploits this production-reproduction duality. The surrogate, who is expected to be a disciplined contract worker who gives up the baby at the termination of the contract, is simultaneously urged to be a nurturing mother for the baby, and a self-less mother who will not negotiate the payment received. The complex interplay of production-reproduction makes the disciplining techniques not just contradictory but also particularly repressive.

When one's identity as a mother is regulated and terminated by a contract, being a good mother often conflicts with being a good worker, which makes it rather difficult to produce the perfect surrogate subject. It requires that this disciplinary project work discursively, through language and metaphor, and physically in the form of dormitory-like surrogacy hostels. By bringing together insights from feminist literature on factory work and global production, I argue that through the various stages of the disciplinary process a new mother-worker subject is produced. At each stage of the disciplinary process, from the recruitment of guilt-ridden mothers to the disciplining of poor, rural, uneducated Indian women, the mother-worker duality is manipulated in ways that most benefit the clinic.

RECRUITING: MANUFACTURING THE PERFECT MOTHER-WORKER SUBJECT

Disciplinary production deploys the art of metaphor, the power of language and the politics of othering and differentiation in crafting a new identity.

—Pun Ngai, *Made in China*

Dr. Usha Khanderia, medical director of the Armaan Maternity Clinic, specializes in infertility and assisted reproductive technologies (ART) like in vitro fertilization, intrauterine insemination, embryo freezing, endoscopic surgeries, and sonography. She had her first successful surrogacy in 2004; in that case the clients arranged for their own surrogate. For her second case, Dr. Khanderia persuaded an employee at her clinic to be a surrogate. Although the ICMR (Indian Council of Medical Research) guidelines specify that the ART center should not be involved with the monetary dealings between the surrogate and the couple or with the recruitment of surrogates, Dr. Khanderia and her crew of nurses and brokers not only recruit the surrogates, but also check the surrogates' medical history, handle the legal paperwork, monitor the surrogates during pregnancy, deliver the babies, and even set up bank accounts for the surrogates to receive their payments from the clients.

Dr. Khanderia recalls her first venture into commercial surrogacy: "An employee in my clinic was our first commercial surrogate. Then through word of mouth her sister-in-law and relatives came in. Gradually we started convincing the women who came to donate eggs. Now there are whole families doing it. We have two families where all the women members are pregnant with someone else's babies. Our nurses convinced them. Not that these women need much convincing."

Dr. Khanderia mentions only two of the three recruitment strategies used by the clinic. The first is through word of mouth, when former surrogates inform their family and friends about surrogacy. Only three of my interviewees heard about surrogacy from former surrogates in their village. This method of spreading the word is limited, since surrogacy is highly stigmatized and most surrogates do not tell their community that they are involved in commercial surrogacy. The second, more successful method of recruitment is to persuade women who come to the clinic for various kinds of treatment to donate eggs in exchange for money (5,000 rupees, or $100) and then recruit them for the more lucrative option—surrogacy. Six of my interviewees followed this path. Dr. Khanderia conveniently glosses over the third recruitment strategy, the most effective of all—formal and informal surrogacy brokers.

At first glance, it might seem surprising that despite the evident poverty in the nearby villages, the clinic needs to devise an active strategy to recruit a sufficient number of women. However, the demographics of the targeted population, mostly people with little education and limited access to media and advertising, imply that the clinic cannot simply wait for the word to spread over time. Brokers also become a critical part of the process because of the high degree of stigma attached to commercial surrogacy in India. Former surrogates, women who could not become surrogates for medical reasons, and midwives, or *dais*, often become brokers. The fluid role of midwives is not unique to Garv. Sarah Pinto, in her detailed ethnography of midwives in a region in North India (2008), reports a similar fluidity in the role of the *dais* or midwives and notes: "Such women are amongst the most mobile in their communities, with intimate knowledge of bodies, reproductive lives, and household histories, as well as a designated, if ambiguous, place in state health schemes" (36). This ambiguous role and intimate knowledge are crucial for the work of brokering within surrogacy. The brokers go from village to village, and door-to-door, to recruit suitable women. Brokers recruited more than half of my interviewees. Vimla, a midwife and broker, brought in nine of the surrogates in this study and charges surrogates up to 10,000 rupees (around $200) each for her services, which might include driving the women to and from the clinic. Vimla describes how she came to be a broker: "I came here to donate eggs but I was refused because of my age. So I started getting women from my hospital. It is easy for me to find the right women because I used to be a midwife. I know which women have very young children, which ones are in desperate need of money."

Recruitment tactics often tap into women's anxiety about being "bad" mothers—mothers who are unable to provide for their children, especially mothers who cannot get their adult daughters married. In India, although fathers are expected to play the breadwinner role, mothers are often castigated by the community for not arranging their daughters' marriages in a timely manner. Regina, one of the oldest surrogates at the clinic, has a teenage daughter with severe mental challenges, and her story exemplifies how fear of being a bad mother affects the decision to become a surrogate: "I came to the clinic when my daughter was ill. The nurse is from my village, and she has seen the state of my daughter. She knows I am old, but she told me if I want to be a surrogate she would try to get me in. I was not agreeing in the beginning. I was too scared. But she said, 'How else will you get that mad daughter of yours married?' "

While Regina became a surrogate to be a good mother for her daughter, Naseem, a 30-year-old surrogate and the mother of a three-year-old boy, heard about surrogacy from the nurses when she came to abort her second pregnancy: "When Jayati [a nurse at the clinic and an informal broker] heard that I am getting the cutting [abortion] done because I can't afford to feed another child, she told me about surrogacy. She told me there is nothing immoral about it, so I agreed."

Naseem, who cannot afford to have her own second child or even feed the first, is instead having a child for someone else to keep. The poignancy of Naseem's reproductive trajectory is just one instance of "stratified reproduction," a term coined by feminist anthropologist Shellee Colen (1995) to describe power relations by which some categories of people are empowered to nurture and reproduce while others are disempowered. Surrogacy in India as an instance of such overt forms of stratified reproduction, or what I classify as neo-eugenics, is analyzed in more detail in chapter 6.

Indeed, by identifying and persuading women who are in desperate need of money to feed, clothe, and educate their own children, the brokers use strategies that rely heavily on the duality of the mother-worker. Being a mother is not just a medical requirement for a woman to be recruited as a surrogate; it is also a mechanism to control her as a worker. This interplay of the mother-worker duality continues to underline the next few steps in the labor process—counseling and the signing of the contract.

COUNSELING AND CONTRACT: MANUFACTURING A PERFECT MOTHER-WORKER MIND

I teach my surrogates one crucial thing: don't treat it like a business; instead, treat it like God's gift to you. Don't be greedy.

—Divya, former surrogate, surrogate counselor, and hostel matron, 2007

Bringing a needy woman from the village to the clinic is a small first step in the whole process. Economic desperation does not make a "perfect" surrogate; she should also be a willing worker and a virtuous mother. The surrogate is expected to be a disciplined contract worker who will give the baby away immediately after delivery without creating a fuss. But she is simultaneously expected to be a nurturing mother, attached to the baby, and a selfless mother who will not treat surrogacy like business. This mother-worker combination is produced through a disciplinary project that deploys the power of language along with a meticulous control over the body of the surrogate. In the next few sections I analyze the discourses used by the medical staff in formal and informal mentoring of surrogates and the language of the contract.

Divya, a former surrogate who is now a surrogate counselor and hostel matron, plays a critical role in disciplining the minds of the surrogates and in the production of a dual mother-worker subject. As a counselor, Divya must inform the surrogates about the entire process, from the embryo transfer to the delivery. But she admits that she uses her discretion when giving the information, especially to the illiterate surrogates.

> My job is to be there for the surrogate—from the date of the transfer to the delivery. What information I give and how I give it depends on the education of the surrogate and her husband. It's not possible to explain everything to them—especially since some of them are totally illiterate. Just yesterday a man came with his wife; he wanted her to become a surrogate. So I started explaining the process to him: "A couple who cannot have a baby of their own will pay you enough money to have a baby for them." The man got up and said, "Okay, I will start tonight. And when my wife is ready [pregnant], I will bring her here." Imagine that! He thought we want *him* to impregnate his wife!

Divya laughs, narrates a few more stories about the ignorance of surrogates and their families, and adds, "Now you see why I don't bother going into the details of the whole process with them?"

After the initial counseling session, the surrogate and her husband have to sign a contract, which specifies their rights (see appendix B). But the form is in English, a language that almost none of the surrogates can read. Divya translates some essential points of the contract for them. So what they do understand is that they have to hand over the baby right after it is born; they have no claims on the baby; neither the doctor nor the couple are responsible for any death resulting from the process; they will receive payments in installments and the last payment will be made after the delivery.

In the words of Gauri, a surrogate, "The only thing they told me was that this thing is not immoral, I will not have to sleep with anyone and that the seed [embryo] will be transferred into me with an injection. They also said that I have to keep the child inside me, rest for the whole time, have medicines on time, and give up the child."

Salma, a surrogate for a couple from Los Angeles, adds, "We were told that if anything happens to the child it's not our responsibility but if anything happens to me, we can't hold anyone responsible. I think the contract says that we will have to give up the child immediately after the delivery—we won't even look at it. Black or white, normal or deformed, we have to give it away."

The inadequate counseling and patronizing attitude toward provision of information has another effect: it further mystifies the unfamiliar technological process for the surrogates. This mystification and subsequent deification of the process and the doctor—the "everyday divine" for surrogates—are explored in chapter 5.

The counseling and the contract (in translation) become critical to the disciplinary process. The contract reiterates the transient role and disposability of the women, not just as workers but also as mothers. This disposability is reiterated at every stage of the process, even though in reality the demand for surrogates is greater than the supply. In other words, there are more couples waiting to hire a surrogate than there are women waiting to be surrogates at the clinic. In fact, a clinic nurse revealed that, as of December 2011, there were more than three hundred intended parents on the waiting list. Concealing, or actively undermining, the true value of surrogates works to the advantage of both the clinic and the client. The nurse and counselor regularly emphasize that the surrogates are merely a vessel; they have no genetic connections with the baby, and it will be taken away from them immediately after delivery. The nurses ensure that the surrogates are not allowed to even breastfeed the baby.[1] These rules, the doctors argue, ensure that the surrogates do not get emotionally attached to the baby and the intended parents face no legal trouble.

Dr. Desai, the only male doctor at the clinic, talks about the ideal profile of a surrogate as compared to the profile of an egg donor:

> We have a different set of priorities for egg donors. In egg donors, we look at the woman's age, intelligence, looks, education, family background etc. For the surrogates it's mostly the character of the womb we are interested in. We make sure the surrogates know that they are not genetically related to the baby, *they are just the wombs* [emphasis added]. But we still have to counsel them a lot before they become ready for surrogacy. It's because of this counseling that we have had no problem with the surrogate not wanting to give the baby up. Our surrogates are not like the surrogates you find in the U.S., who feign attachment just to make some extra bucks. This is one of the big reasons why we get so many international clients.

According to Dr. Desai, then, the counseling session reiterates the transient nature of the surrogate's mothering role. The surrogate mother is told that she is merely a womb; this is meant to prevent her from getting emotionally attached to the baby. It also underscores her disposability as a worker, discouraging her from "feigning" attachment to the baby in order to negotiate higher wages.

Dr. Khanderia, the chief doctor and proprietor of the clinic, has a slightly different take on the qualities required from a surrogate:

> I have to educate them about everything because all these women are poor and illiterate villagers. I tell them, "You have to do nothing. It's not your baby. You are just providing it a home in your womb for nine months because it doesn't have a house of its own. If some child comes to stay with you for just nine months what will you do? You will take care of it even more, love it even more than you love your own, because it is someone else's. This is the same thing. You will take care of the baby for nine months and then give it to its mother. And for that you will be paid." I think, *finally, how you train them—that is what makes surrogacy work* [emphasis added].

Dr. Khanderia's "training" of first-time surrogates reiterates the disposability of the woman-womb but adds the contradictory demand that the surrogate be nurturing toward the baby and yet detached from it.[2]

Her comments reveal the complex mother-worker combination demanded from a surrogate, to simultaneously be a temporary yet professional caretaker and a nurturing mother. The perfect surrogate is one who is constantly aware of her disposability and the transience of her identity as a worker and yet loves the product of her transient labor (the fetus) as her own.

Although contracts indicate the actual remuneration, in the absence of any binding law, individual intended parents have considerable freedom in deciding the final amount. Payments made to the surrogate range from as low as $2,000 to as much as $8,000. The base rate had gone up by the time of my third visit to the field, and most women reported receiving at least $4,000. But differential rates remain the norm, and the final amount is often determined by the generosity of individual clients. The payment is made in three installments, one when the pregnancy is confirmed, the second after the second trimester, and the final amount after delivery. Most surrogates and their husbands have at least one meeting with the intended parents before the embryo transfer. The length and frequency of these meetings depend on the intended parents. Most intended parents from India continue to meet with the surrogates throughout the pregnancy, while many international couples meet the surrogate once before the embryo transfer and again at the time of delivery.

Surrogates are typically expected to stay at the clinic or at one of the surrogacy hostels after the embryo transfer. The intended parents pay for the monthly maintenance of the surrogates, a cost that ranges from $20 to $100 per month. Surrogates undergoing caesarean sections are allowed to rest and recover at the clinic or the hostel. The length of the recovery period at the clinic depends on the willingness of the couple to pay for the extended stay, and the health of the surrogate after the delivery. During this entire process, Divya also acts as a mediator for surrogates who are uneducated or can't speak English but have international clients.

Although Divya serves as an intermediary between the surrogates and their clients, her loyalties seem to be ambiguous. On the one hand, being a former surrogate and sharing living space with the surrogates makes Divya a mentor and guide for them. As a hostel matron, Divya occasionally becomes a champion of surrogates' rights, conveying their demands and complaints to the doctor and the clients. On the other hand, Divya's class background and her ability to converse in English position her closer to the clients. Divya's loyalty toward the medical staff and the intended parents is revealed in her informal counseling sessions with the surrogates in the hostel. Although she wants the couples hiring surrogates to get the best business deal possible, she disapproves of surrogates' negotiating their wages: "My task is to make sure that the clients don't get fooled—they get the best deal possible. After all, they are investing so much money in my surrogates. Of course, I also want the best deal for the surrogates. I know how painful this thing is. I have been there myself. But I teach my surrogates one crucial thing: Don't treat it like a business; instead, treat it like God's gift to you. *Don't be greedy.*"

Divya's statement reflects the ambiguity surrounding commercial surrogacy: it lies somewhere between contractual labor and motherly altruism.[3] But interestingly, this ambiguity works differently for buyers and sellers of surrogacy. While Divya recognizes the business aspect of surrogacy and the "investment" made by the buyers of this labor (the intended parents), she simultaneously instructs the sellers (the surrogates) to treat it like God's gift, the underlying instruction being not to negotiate the wages. Previous scholarship on surrogacy in the global north, especially in North America, indicates that surrogacy program managers often construct surrogates as "gift-giving angels" to soften the pecuniary image of commercial surrogacy (Ragone 1994). Oddly, although Divya evokes the gift metaphor in the narrative above, she uses it in a very different way—in her interpretation, surrogacy is *God's* gift to needy mothers. God gives Indian (surrogate) mothers an opportunity to fulfill their familial duties. While the surrogate in other contexts chooses to give a gift to the intended parents, God makes the choices for Indian surrogates.[4]

Vimla, a broker and matron of another surrogacy hostel, conducts her counseling sessions a little differently from the way Divya conducts hers. Vimla says:

> To convince the women I often explain to them that it's like renting a house for a year. We want to rent your womb for a year, and Doctor Madam will get you money in return. I tell them surrogacy is not immoral. It is much better than a woman going from one man's bed to the next to make money. Here she earns 2 lakhs [$5,000] and that will keep her going for at least three years. Prostitution will not pay her that much and can also lead to diseases.

Vimla stresses the business aspect of surrogacy by using the metaphor of renting a house and by comparing surrogacy to prostitution. Although she understands the technology of surrogacy, she uses the surrogate-prostitute analogy, which is often used by people who are not familiar with assisted reproductive technology. The surrogate-prostitute comparison plays a critical role in the disciplinary project. It is simultaneously challenged and reinforced by the brokers, counselors, and medical professionals at different stages of the labor process. At the time of recruitment and counseling, the surrogates are assured that their role does not involve any immoral acts like sleeping with clients. In informal counseling and mentoring sessions, however, the "bad" surrogate is often compared to a prostitute. Consequently, the surrogate is under constant fear of crossing the thin line between morality and immorality and disturbing the delicate balance of being a perfect mother-worker.

While sipping tea with some surrogates at her hostel, Divya criticizes Vimla and her brokering style:

> I don't know where Vimla gets her women. You know what I call her, a dirty *bharhwa* [pimp]. She never tries to find out about the family of the surrogate. For all you know she gets prostitutes. It's criminal what she does to the trust of the intended parents. They trust their lives on this surrogate and if she turns out to be a prostitute, then their baby will grow in a dirty womb. She once got a "loose" woman [prostitute] who delivered babies to her clients and then eloped with another surrogate's husband! No one here has any respect for such brokers or the women she brings.[5]

What makes a good surrogate versus a bad surrogate is often talked about in counseling sessions and at informal lectures in the hostels, and new residents are encouraged to stay away from bad influences like "greedy" Vimla and the immoral surrogates she brings to the clinic and hostel. Divya lectures her surrogates:

> I don't want any of you to behave like surrogate Puja [a surrogate brought to the clinic by Vimla], treating this like a moneymaking business and manipulating the nice couple from America. Whenever I meet Puja or that broker Vimla I feel like saying, "First start taking care of your own children." Such dirty clothes Puja's boy wears and his nose is always running. And who knows who Vimla's daughter is sleeping with. She hangs around with ten boys at the same time.

Puja and Vimla are depicted as bad models for the surrogates because they are not just greedy workers (prostitutes or pimps) but also unfit mothers. Puja is incapable of being a good surrogate, a caretaker of someone else's child, since she is not a good mother to her own children. To be a perfect surrogate, a woman has to be a good mother first and then a good contract worker.

The counseling sessions and the various metaphors used thus become a critical tool in the disciplinary project. The discourse of disposability emphasizes detachment from the child and keeps the negotiating power of the surrogates in check. An egg donor with special characteristics could negotiate a higher price, but a womb like any other womb is waiting to be hired by a client. The demand for professionalism ensures that the surrogate hands over the baby without causing any trouble for the clients. The professional surrogate, however, cannot be business-minded. She is to treat surrogacy as an opportunity to fulfill her duties as a mother. Moreover, the disciplinary project not only emphasizes a perfect worker model but also demands perfect mother qualities from the surrogates. A good surrogate loves the product of her transient labor as her own. Good mothering qualities are required not just in conjunction with the good worker qualities but independently as well. A surrogate has to be a good mother to her own child before she can be a mother-worker for someone else's baby.

The contract and the counseling constitute the first step in the disciplinary process. The surrogates in Garv are desirable not just because they are cheap but also because they are fully under the control of the doctor and the buyer. To ensure that the women remain perfect surrogates and the clients get the best deal, the management has devised a way to have complete control over the surrogates during the nine months of pregnancy: surrogacy hostels.

SURROGACY HOSTELS: MANUFACTURING A PERFECT MOTHER-WORKER BODY

What was so new about these projects of docility . . . ? [An] uninterrupted, constant coercion, supervising the process of the activity rather than its result; and it is exercised according to a codification that partitions as closely as possible time, space, movement.

—Michel Foucault, *Discipline and Punish*

Scholars writing on gender and factory work have demonstrated how dormitory techniques of power are central to the extraction of labor from workers.[6] The underlying principle of the dormitory system is not just to impose severe discipline and surveillance but also to create a constant need for self-discipline and internalized surveillance. In this section I demonstrate how the surrogacy hostel and clinic, the use of timetables, and the practice of ranking surrogates, as well as the subtle self-supervision of everyday lives, are used to create the perfect mother-worker.

Surrogates typically have two kinds of living arrangements during their months of pregnancy: living in the rooms above the clinic under Dr. Khanderia's care or living in the hostels financed by the clinic. The doctors decide whether an individual will go from one to the other during her pregnancy. These living arrangements are the least discreet of the disciplinary techniques used by the clinic, by which the surrogates can literally be kept under constant surveillance. In the clinic, the surrogates live in groups of eight to a room. The rooms are lined with single iron beds, with barely enough space to walk between them. One end of the beds is kept raised with a wooden block so that the surrogate can have her legs up after the embryo transfer. Most rooms have pictures of happy babies and an infant Lord Krishna (a Hindu god), clothes hanging from a makeshift clothesline, and a few extra chairs for visitors. The women have nothing to do the whole day except pace up and down on the same floor. They are not allowed to climb the stairs, and they have to wait for the nurses to operate the elevator. They talk with one another, sharing their woes and experiences, as they wait for the next injection or pill. As Sheela Saravanan (2010, 27) notes in her commentary on the lives of 13 surrogates in two clinics in India, "inertness and submissiveness" are the primary disciplinary requirements in the hostels.

The surrogacy hostels, located in towns close to the clinic, are less sterile, and the surrogates have fewer restrictions on their movement. They have access to a kitchen (along with a cook), a television, and a prayer room. Husbands are allowed to visit but are encouraged not to stay the night, to emphasize the requirement that the surrogate cannot have any sexual relations during the nine months of pregnancy. The hostels are spaces where the daily activities of the surrogates can be not just monitored but also controlled. The timetable establishes a rhythm that is meant to ensure a healthy and docile mother-worker. Varsha is a surrogate for a couple from Uttar Pradesh, India. She lists the daily schedule for the surrogates at the clinic:

> Get up at 8 am and have some vitamins with our tea and breakfast. Sleep. Get up in time for Doctor Madam's visit or the nurse's injections, for those who still need injections. Sleep. Get up for lunch. Mostly we get served a fixed lunch, along with whatever medicines we have left. The doctor wants me to eat too much here. I enjoyed it in the beginning but now sometimes I feel like I would burst! Madam has told us that all mothers who want a healthy baby should take this diet. I know it's required for the baby so I can't create a fuss.

The surrogates are instructed to take the diet that all responsible mothers should take for their babies' good health. Their duty as a responsible mother is underscored not just as a disciplinary technique but also as an incentive. Varsha explains: "I am being extra careful now because Doctor Madam has said if everything looks all right in the ultrasound I can go visit my children. I don't want to do anything that will make Madam change her mind about letting me go home for a day or two."

For Varsha and other surrogates with young children, the promise of being able to see their own children, "if everything went well," serves as an ever-present incentive to follow instructions and be the perfect mother-worker. Here the contradictory demands made on the perfect mother-worker are stark—while "bad" surrogates are constantly being chastised for not taking care of their children, the surrogacy arrangement requires that the good (disciplined) worker stay willingly at the clinic, away from her family and her children.

The surrogates living in the hostels away from the clinic have a less rigid schedule and more leisure activities. However, the leisure activities are engineered to make them better workers in this round of pregnancy or the next: classes in English that would enable the surrogate to converse with her international client and report her daily health and activities, and computer lessons to facilitate further communication with international clients.

Tina, a surrogate for a couple from Dubai, thinks the hostel feels like home despite the rules and injections, perhaps because of these leisure activities: "This doesn't feel like a hostel at all. This is more like home. As long as we are inside the house we can move around freely, watch TV, sleep. We even have a prayer room where we all pray in the mornings and evenings."

Detailed regulation of the surrogates' private time allows prolonged control in a way that is not possible when there is a separation between home and work. Regulation of the surrogates' leisure time also reinforces the perfect mother-worker identity. The computer and English lessons create a better worker (for now and the future), who can communicate more effectively with the couple hiring her, while the elaborate prayer room and scheduled prayer hours emphasize the image of a virtuous, religious, and docile mother-worker.

The metaphors of hostel as home and training as leisure not only dilute the labor aspect of surrogacy but are used to justify the surveillance of surrogates. As Dr. Desai argues:

> In a way it's also very good for all the mothers to stay together, laugh, play and stay happy. It's a good way of passing time for them. And it prevents them from always wanting to go home. If we send her home, she is bound to start doing housework. *She doesn't know any better.* But here we can ensure that she gets complete rest. When the surrogate has her own children, she has it without even realizing what happened—in fun and games. But in this pregnancy a lot depends on her actions. And we want nothing to go wrong. In the other hostel, we've also started English and computer lessons for them. We want them to learn something, some skills to face the world better after staying with us. *We can't take care of them forever!* [emphasis added]

Dr. Desai's comments reiterate the need to modernize the women. The untrained mothers need to be kept in the hostel because they cannot be expected to understand the modern methods of motherhood. Interestingly, Dr. Desai also argues that the hostel is both a haven for the surrogates and a place where they will be trained to face the real world. Scholars of work, especially in global production and factories, have discussed the paternalistic tropes that managers use to justify the surveillance of women workers as well as to emphasize the temporary and secondary nature of their employment. The factory workers in this context are young, unmarried women, employed mostly for a brief period before marriage. Ironically, Dr. Desai uses a similar paternalistic narrative for the surrogates, who are married women with children. Here the paternalism stems from the assumed illiteracy of these women, their inexperience with modern methods of motherhood and technologies, and their assumed unfamiliarity with the public space of "real work."

The blurring of the home with the work space further reiterates the dual mother-worker role demanded from the surrogates; while the hostel becomes a space of refuge where they eat, pray, and engage in recreation like responsible mothers, it is also the place where they are trained to be better workers. Dr. Desai's assumption about the women's housewife status and inability to deal with the real world is ironic, since only a third of the surrogates identify as housewives. Their presumed housewife status further underscores their primary role as mothers and wives, rather than as workers. Moreover, the surrogates are portrayed as not just untrained workers but also untrained mothers. The English and computer classes, as well as the women's living arrangements, are meant to "modernize" these women, replacing traditional forms of mothering with what the doctor believes to be Western, upper-class, and "healthy" forms of pregnancy and mothering. The clinic is thus training the women to be good mothers—fit to produce children for their "modern" clients.

The disciplinary machinery, however, works in a more detailed way than just enclosing the surrogates in hostels. Surrogates are organized into ranks: the first are surrogates recovering from embryo transfer, those who are awaiting confirmation of pregnancy, or those who are in their first months of pregnancy. These women are usually kept in a small room at the clinic under close surveillance. They are actively disciplined to be docile workers—rest, eat, and take injections and medicines on time. The anxiety in this room is always high and the surrogates in the next room are looked at with envy as ones who have successfully passed the first trimester. The surrogates in the second, bigger room have confirmed pregnancies, usually in their second or last trimester. The atmosphere is more relaxed and the surrogates are allowed to roam freely on that floor of the clinic. The quiet hours for this room are only after lunch and dinner, and these surrogates are allowed more visits from their families.

As the surrogates move up in rank, the emphasis moves from disciplinary rules to more subtle surveillance and an emphasis on self-supervision of everyday lives and daily activities. While the first-time surrogates and women in their first trimester are given medicine and injections by nurses, the surrogates at the hostel outside the clinic and repeat surrogates are encouraged to self-monitor their medicines, injections, food, and rest. As Divya summarizes:

> With my girls there is no tension. I keep them like it's their house. It's not like a hostel with restriction on food, activity or movement. I tell them right at the beginning that if you treat this like someone else's house then

you would find it very hard to be happy in the months away from your family. I urge them to be self-sufficient, take responsibility, go cook in the kitchen whenever they like. By now they should have learnt what they can do without harming the baby. I should not have to tell them anything.

The paradoxical portrayal of gestation and pregnancy as being "natural" for women as well as being something that requires "training" necessitates these different forms of discipline in the hostel—from explicit surveillance of different ranks to meticulous self-supervision of everyday lives. Unlike Dr. Desai's depiction of surrogates as vulnerable and untrained mothers, Divya's narrative encourages the surrogates to behave like self-disciplined, responsible mothers who know how to take care of the baby growing inside them.

The surrogates recovering from delivery, especially those who are recovering from a caesarean section, constitute the third rank. These surrogates—often weak from surgery and emotional after giving the baby away—are kept on a separate floor and allowed to recuperate. The surrogates who are still pregnant typically get news about whether it was a boy or a girl from the nurses, but interaction between current and departing surrogates is actively discouraged.

Apart from ranking and partitioning based on trimester and stage of pregnancy, there is an additional partitioning—placing some surrogates in the clinic instead of the hostels. "Problem" surrogates are often kept in the clinic, under the doctor's constant supervision. These surrogates are either women who require maximum medical attention, such as those carrying twins or triplets, older surrogates, or those who require maximum surveillance because of their personality. Regina is clearly a "problem" surrogate, not just because of her age but also because of her insubordinate disposition. Regina claims that she is 40 years old, but she looks much older, and the doctors suspect that her broker has provided a fake birth certificate. Regina regularly tries to sneak out of the clinic to check on her sick daughter. Hostel matron and counselor Divya complains about Regina:

> She is good at heart but she is just not suited for this, she is too old, *too set in her ways.* She just does not want to stay inside the room, forget about lying in bed. Did you see how she sauntered out of the elevator with no care? She doesn't seem to understand that she is 45 years old and over 30 weeks pregnant! I know she wanted to move into my hostel but I said "No!" There was no way I want to be responsible for her.

Not surprisingly, Regina, a deviant worker who is too "set in her ways" to be molded like the rest, remained confined to the clinic until the date of her delivery.

The final form of ranking is, curiously, based not on the characteristics of the surrogates but on the nationality of the couple hiring them. This is the most pronounced form of ranking at the clinic. The surrogates of foreign couples are allotted the "luxury" rooms. This is partly because the intended parents often visit their surrogates during late pregnancy. The term "foreign" excludes anyone of Indian origin and surrogates hired by non-resident Indians. Only surrogates hired by "real foreigners" (anyone who is not Indian or of Indian origin) are assigned the luxury rooms.[7] The number of luxury rooms, however, is limited, and the privileged few surrogates hired by "real foreigners" are transferred to these rooms only during their last trimester. There is a stark difference between the general rooms and the luxury rooms. While a general room has minimal furniture—eight to ten iron cots, a shared bathroom, and barely any comforts—the luxury room is equipped with a color television, air conditioner, and attached bath. Neeti, a nurse at the clinic, justifies the ranking by saying: "We have to do at least this much for our foreign clients. In any case these surrogates deserve this. They are at the last stage and have successfully kept the pregnancy."

When I interrupt her and ask why all surrogates in the last trimester are not rewarded in a similar fashion, Neeti shrugs and replies: "Right from start the ones hired by foreign couples have it better—whether it be tips, cell phone or small gifts. In any case they all have to go back and stay in their own homes where, forget AC, some don't even have fans! The girls [surrogates] know all this and they don't complain. They are happy with whatever they get. As a matter of fact, some feel more isolated in these [luxury] rooms."

According to Neeti, the luxury rooms are a reward reserved for surrogates of international couples, and the other, less-privileged surrogates accept this hierarchy. Presumably another virtue of the perfect mother-worker, trained not to be business-minded and greedy, is to accept all material benefits as non-negotiable gifts. I consider the construction of surrogates as needy gift-receivers in more detail in chapter 5.

I want to pause at this juncture and recognize the dilemmas I often face as a feminist researcher of a new and intensely provocative form of labor. Despite my conscious effort to avoid potentially orientalist frames, I realize that many first-time readers of my work are horrified by the disciplinary project, especially the hostel arrangements devised by the doctor and her associates. Inadvertently, description of the disciplinary tactics conjures up the exact images that I wanted to challenge when I started this project. It might be constructive at this stage to recognize that although at first glance the disciplinary project appears to be uncanny, discomforting, and almost like science fiction, it is in fact not that unusual. Workers in factories and in assembly-line production, especially women workers residing in dormitories attached to such factories, are subjected to a similar disciplinary regimen. Earlier in the chapter I mentioned the parallels between the paternalistic disciplinary tropes used by the clinic and those devised by factory managers. Other scholars of factory labor discipline have written at length about new technologies of power where Taylorism, or extreme labor discipline and supervision of work, is complemented by techniques that operate through the continual surveillance of space and the bodies (and bodily movements) of workers. These disciplinary procedures often include close monitoring of workers' bodies: for instance, management monitoring the appearance and dress code of women workers, their daily activities, relationships and sexual activities, and even toilet breaks (Freeman 2000; Ngai 2000; Ong 1987). Hostels for pregnant women may make us queasy, but such residential surveillance techniques have precedents in the past, whether in the form of early mill towns in New England that provided housing and "oversight" for newly recruited workers or, more recently, the dormitory system encountered in many factories in Asia (Dublin 1975; Ong 1987; Ngai 2000; Wright 2006). In her insightful work on surrogate mothers in Bangalore, sociologist Sharmila Rudrappa (2012) compares the life of women in "Bangalore's reproduction industry" to a common alternative source of livelihood in that region—working in a garment factory, for instance—and argues that surrogacy allows women "the possibility of extracting greater value from their bodies once they have been deemed unproductive workers in garment factories" (22). On the basis of the life history of the protagonist in her study, a former garment factory worker, Rudrappa persuasively argues that the surveillance of the surrogacy hostel was almost "benign in comparison to the surveillance and punishment meted out for supposed infractions on the garment shop floor, where long conversations with teammates, taking a few minutes of rest, or going on breaks were all curtailed" (24).

Much like the physical space of surveillance, the managerial discourse—whether it be the stigmatizing discourse of surrogates as prostitutes or the contradictory portrayal of gestation as natural for women as well as something that requires surveillance—resonates with managerial tactics in other gendered forms of work. Invoking "stigma" and "nature" seems to be a popular labor control mechanism, especially for women workers. In their book *Intimate Labors: Cultures Technologies, and the Politics of Care* (2007), sociologists Eileen Boris and Rhacel Salazar Parreñas speak of the "devaluation thesis" in all forms of *intimate* labor—labor like care work, sex work, and domestic work (7). The conflation of intimate labor with love (the myth of "labor of love") or family obligation has historically justified lower wages. When intimacy becomes labor, it becomes regarded as unskilled work that anyone can perform because women have performed these activities historically without pay. This, Boris and Parreñas argue, leads to a "double devaluation" because of the lack of pay and the "nature" of doers. This devaluation based on the naturalization of skills is not restricted to intimate forms of labor. For instance, there is much evidence that transnational capitalism produces discourses that naturalize the subordination of women *factory* workers. Management often justifies its preference for women workers in the global south by using the twin rhetoric of nimble fingers and innate docility. For instance, Collins (2002) demonstrates how managers in an apparel industry in North America construe the offshore women workers as "natural resources" who were born with and had not acquired the skills required. Like their Mexican sisters born with the innate ability to sew, the surrogates in Garv presumably have the innate ability to procreate and thus can be paid less than their counterparts in the global north.

While naturalization of skills effectively *cheapens* women's labor, stigmatization of labor efficiently *controls* women's labor. Again, this rhetoric of stigma is not limited to sex work or surrogacy. Throughout industrializing Asia and Mexico, as young women become the rapidly growing new workforce and engage in activities that violate traditional boundaries in public life (much like the production-reproduction boundary violated by commercial surrogates), they are disciplined by the rhetoric of stigma and shame. In Malaysia, for example, the influx of young rural women into industrial sites is considered the cause of the moral decadence in Malay-Muslim societies, where Malay working women are perceived as an "Other invading male public spaces," the "Other" that needs to be controlled (Ong 1987, 287). In South India, this taint carries over to care work, with nurses being stigmatized as lower-class, sexually loose women with too much independence (George 2000). Whether used for factory workers, care workers, or migrant domestic workers, the "dirty worker" label seems to be a common strategy of control (Anderson 1990; Cole and Booth 2007; George 2000). Chapter 6 explores the narratives and strategies of surrogates as they negotiate these stigmatizing and disciplinary discourses.

This chapter focused on the disciplinary project—the production of the "mother-worker" subject. In the absence of any other in-depth work on surrogacy in India, it is as important to first scrutinize the nature and structures of domination as it is to highlight the creative strategies employed by surrogates to negotiate or subvert these relationships of power. The resistive strategies of the surrogates, in essence, explicate the complex web of power relations. At various stages of the surrogacy process, the surrogates negotiate with the family and the clinic to gain control over their own bodies and reproductive futures. These negotiations are in response to the disciplinary tactics used by the clinic and in response to the medical construction of surrogates as dirty workers and disposable mothers. Although these negotiations are ostensibly at the micro political level, they are notably affected by and have repercussions at the macro level, namely at the level of the state. Simultaneously, they often speak to the unequal power relationships between the buyers and the sellers of surrogacy—inequalities based on race, class, and citizenship.

5 ✌ EVERYDAY DIVINITIES AND GOD'S LABOR

You talk about Hindu-Muslim-Christian. Those are gods for the educated. But it is different for all of us, this surro-dev [Surro-god] made this all possible for us. . . . These are our two gods [she points to the pictures on the wall]: Lord Krishna [a Hindu god] and Doctor Devi [Doctor Goddess].

—Tina, a Christian surrogate living in a surrogacy hostel, 2007

This is my mission and I am grateful that I can be a part of this divine intervention to change two sets of lives.

—Dr. Usha Khanderia, Armaan Maternity Clinic, 2007

What really helped us take this decision was that we knew our surrogate wouldn't spend the money for drugs or a flat-screen TV. She would be using it to feed her family, build her own house. . . . I am not religious, but this seemed almost like God's work, call it a worthy cause . . . a mission.

—Judy, intended mother from the United States,
Armaan Maternity Clinic, 2008

THIS CHAPTER was exceptionally hard to write. The reason is partly personal—I have an uncomfortable relationship with institutionalized or organized religion, and to whatever extent possible, I avoid public conversations about divinity. This ironically worked out well for me, as I was advised ahead of my fieldwork trip to avoid unprovoked discussions about religion in this region of India, where extreme forms of Hindu nationalism have wreaked havoc in the past decade. The lingering effect of the brutal and systematic carnage of a minority community is palpable in the environment of fear that persists to this day.[1] But after careful analysis of the transcribed conversations that I held over the course of my stay in Garv, I realized that narratives of the divine, when used by those involved in surrogacy at the clinic, have little to do with organized religion.

For the surrogates at Armaan clinic and hostel, what I call the "everyday divine" takes precedence over organized religion. The process of surrogacy and the doctor herself are deified, while religious endogamy and prescriptions are underplayed. But apart from constructing such creative forms of divinity, the narratives of divinity were startling on another front. Previous ethnographies of surrogacy in other parts of the world have revealed that surrogates often construct the surrogate birth as their divine gift to the intended parents, and themselves as angels and messengers of God (Ragone 1994; Teman 2010). In my conversations with the surrogates, the glaring absence of the gift-giving narrative was hard to miss and equally hard to explain.

SURROGACY AND THE DIVINE IN INDIA

Religious perspectives on assisted conception and reproductive technologies shape not just discussions on bioethics but also the cultural tools available to users of these technologies for meaning-making. I devote the first section of this chapter to reflections on assisted conception within Hinduism, in part because the majority of my respondents—surrogates, brokers, and doctors—identified as Hindu. But the popularity of characters from Hindu epics and mythology cuts across religions, and women, irrespective of their religion, evoked narratives from Hindu mythology to make sense of their involvement in surrogacy. A brief sketch of some relevant parables provides fascinating insight into the "traditional" idioms available to actors for making sense of the "modern" practice of surrogacy. These idioms keep surfacing, not just in this chapter but in the rest of the book as well.

Hinduism is widely accepted as being far more flexible about assisted conception than Christianity, Judaism, or Islam.[2] But this flexibility does not arise from a lack of discussion and debate on assisted conception (Kumar 2007). In fact, the variety of ancient Hindu parables that focus on assisted conception is quite remarkable. There are detailed and numerous discussions on "strategies of heirship" in the Hindu epic *Mahabharata*, many of which involve creative ways of procreation (Sutherland 1990). For instance, the stories in this epic of the three queens, Kunti, Madri, and Gandhari, as they struggle to overcome challenges of infertility reflect very early discussions on assisted conception. One such creative practice interwoven into this epic is that of *niyoga* (sometimes referred to as male surrogacy), the appointment of a (surrogate) man to impregnate the wife and enable the procreation of a son and heir.[3] Surrogacy, in various guises, appears to be a popular theme in Hindu mythology, especially in tales involving demon King Kansa. According to the epic *Bhagvata Purana*, Kansa was intent upon killing all of his sister's children because of a prediction that he would die at the hands of her eighth son. Kansa threw his sister, Devaki, and her husband, Vasudeva, in prison and proceeded to kill their first six children. Lord Vishnu heard his disciple Vasudeva's prayers and miraculously transferred the seventh embryo from Devaki's womb to the womb of Rohini (Vasudeva's second wife). Rohini gave birth to the baby and secretly raised the child. But surrogate mother Rohini is not as celebrated as the other surrogate mother in the same tale—Yashoda. Vasudeva's eighth child, Krishna, who was predicted to meet the same fate as his first six siblings, was secretly exchanged for a cowherd's daughter. Lord Krishna was brought up by the cowherd's wife, Yashoda, and most stories surrounding Lord Krishna in his infant years are about the loving bond shared between him and his "surrogate" or foster mother, Yashoda. This mother-son interaction is a popular theme in media representations of Indian mythology, as well as in Hindu devotional songs and prayers. Innumerable devotional songs have been dedicated to establishing Yashoda's loyal motherhood, in which Yashoda bathes and dresses the child, cooks for him, feeds him, tells him stories, and rocks him to sleep (Krishnan 1990). Not surprisingly, the surrogates regularly invoke this particular mother-son relationship. These mythological characters allow surrogates to reimagine kinship ties with the baby and resist the medical construction of surrogates as disposable mothers.

But idioms of divine evoked every day at the clinic are not restricted to mythological characters. In the narratives of the surrogates, the process of surrogacy is sacralised and Dr. Khanderia becomes a demigoddess on a par with Lord Krishna.

SURRO-*DEV* AND USHA DEVI: SURROGATES AND THE "EVERYDAY DIVINE"

It is six o'clock in the evening, prayer hour for the surrogates in Divya's hostel, but most of the surrogates remain glued to the television set watching a family drama in Hindi. Tina, Mansi, and Naseem lead me to the prayer room, a small but brightly decorated space in the hostel. In one corner is a small collection of Hindu idols, and the walls are plastered with bright pictures of many more Hindu gods and goddesses. Sharda, another surrogate at the hostel, has covered her head with a *dupatta* (stole) and is chanting softly. We sit behind her as Naseem, one of two Muslims in the hostel, and Tina, a convert to Christianity, enthusiastically join in the chanting.

After prayer, I ask Naseem why she participates in a Hindu praying session. Naseem and Tina laugh loudly at my query and drag me to their beds on one side of the dormitory. Here the walls are bare except for a popular Anne Geddes calendar picture of laughing Caucasian babies popping out of pumpkins, a picture of Lord Krishna, and a newspaper cutting of a beaming Dr. Khanderia. Tina points to the pictures on the wall and introduces me to Usha *devi*, one of two "everyday divinities" and a popular demigoddess for the surrogates at the clinic.

> We [Tina and her husband] are from a Christian community. All our neighbors are Christians and we all go to Church every Sunday. But here [for surrogates], things are different. These are our two Gods: Lord Krishna [a Hindu God] and Doctor *devi* [Doctor Goddess]. Yes, we are Christians, my husband is a very good Christian. But I grew up hearing stories of Lord Krishna. Divya *didi* [the matron] tells us that even Doctor Madam worships him. . . . You can say Madam is our real *Devi*. We don't see her often but she comes to check on our health sometimes. But Divya *didi* talks about her all the time.

For Tina, a practicing Christian, Christianity is on hold. While she is at the hostel, the doctor as well as the God (Lord Krishna) worshipped by the doctor and by her colleagues take precedence over Christianity. Naseem, another surrogate who belongs to a minority religion, talks about her dilemma as a Muslim surrogate:

> It is hard for me, you know, being a Muslim. I am not sure, but I think we [Muslims] are not allowed to do this [become a surrogate]. I am not going to tell anyone in my community. But Doctor Madam says there is nothing wrong with what I am doing. She knows so much, why should I not believe her? She says this will change our lives. She has helped so many women, you know. There are pictures on the walls—she has helped women from Africa, America, abroad. She is a miracle woman. She is our *devi*.

Naseem's anxiety about her religion not approving of her decision to become a surrogate is eased by the "miracle" doctor. Surrogates at the clinic are not unusual in their reverence for the doctor. Doctors have conventionally been viewed and revered as life-giving, miracle-working gods in India. This deification gets amplified in situations of death and birth. For instance, researchers on infertility in India have noticed such narratives of reverence among patients seeking infertility treatment and their construction of clinicians as "demi-gods of fertility" (Bharadwaj 2000, 461). Doctors report the "blind faith" of their patients—their belief in the doctor's ability to perform miracles—rather than faith in the effectiveness of technology and medicine. For surrogates at the hostel, the reverence for Dr. Khanderia is, in part, also due to the mystique surrounding her. As Tina reports, the doctor is an infrequent visitor to the hostel, but her accomplishments are narrated time and again by matron Divya. There was a buzz of excitement every time the doctor visited the hostel: this was the surrogates' opportunity to have direct interactions with their *devi*, unmediated by the matron. I experienced this aura and mystery surrounding her as well. During my entire stay, my interactions with the doctor were minimal, and my requests for appointments usually left to fate. "No one knows when she will be free, she is out on her rounds" was the typical response by the nurses.

Later in the conversation, Tina and Sharda introduce me to another innovative addition to the divine—surro-*dev* (surro-god). This was the first time I heard the word "surro-*dev*," but over the course of my fieldwork, I heard it repeatedly from surrogates and their husbands. Was this word simply a distortion by the surrogates of the unfamiliar English word "surrogacy"? I ask Tina why she combines "surro" with the Hindi word *dev* (god). She seems surprised by the naïveté of my question:

> You talk about Hindu-Muslim-Christian. Those are Gods for the educated. But it is like this for all of us, this surro-*dev* [surro-god] made this all possible for us. Where was I before this? Where was she [Sharda]? My husband is an auto-rickshaw driver, but he does not own the rickshaw and I have four children to feed. I heard about surro-*dev* from my sister-in-law. *I do not understand what it is, but I know it makes impossible things possible* [emphasis added] for us.

Tina echoes another claim made by several surrogates: religious endogamy is for the educated, and these categories become fluid within the surrogacy hostels. The kinship ties forged by surrogates that (temporarily) traverse boundaries of religious endogamy are discussed in chapter 7. Curiously, the surrogates who belong to minority communities—Muslims and Christians—most actively evoke such alternative forms of divinity. Although these respondents were unsure about the acceptability of surrogacy within their religion, they intuitively predicted that such processes would be prohibited. Surrogate Razia summarized the situation perfectly when she announced: "I don't want to know what the Quran says about this. Isn't it better this way?"

The reverence for surrogacy in Tina's narrative, much like the deification of the doctor, can be linked to the mystification of the process. This mystification is a result of the disciplinary project—the counseling and the contract (see chapter 4). Tina does not understand what surrogacy really entails, and this unfamiliar, unexplained technology, which could potentially change her life, becomes her god. Betsy Hartmann, in her groundbreaking book *Reproductive Rights and Wrongs: The Global Politics of Population Control*, spoke of the "injection mystique" existing in many areas of the global south, especially in areas that are exposed to low levels of biomedicalization. People associated injections with safe, effective medicine, and were eager to receive them (Hartmann 1995, 201). But this inherent faith in injections made it easier to administer injections, even long-term, controversial injectibles like Depo-Provera, without explaining the side effects. The surrogates' reverence for the surrogacy process and the doctor resonates with the "injections mystique." It ensures that the surrogates do not question the grossly inadequate explanation of the medical aspects of surrogacy and its physiological effects and risks.

The disciplining project shapes the interplay of divinity and surrogacy in yet another way as well. While surrogates in other parts of the world depict themselves as "angels giving the ultimate gift of God," the disciplined surrogates of India construct surrogacy as God's gift to poor and needy mothers.

SURROGATES AS ANGELS AND PREGNANT FAIRIES

Metaphors like "the child as an ultimate gift of God" and the surrogate as a "pregnant fairy" or "an angel sent by God" are rampant in academic literature, women's narratives, and online forums on surrogacy in the global north. Such metaphors are often evoked by surrogates, intended mothers, and surrogacy programs to soften the pecuniary image of commercial surrogacy (Ragone 1994; Raymond 1990, 1993; Teman 2010). In her study of surrogates in the United States, Ragone shows that surrogates consistently denied that receiving remuneration is their primary motivation and instead emphasized their desire to give "the ultimate gift of love" (1994, 59). According to feminist activist and social scientist Janice Raymond (1990), this "dominance of altruism and gift-giving as an ethical norm in the global north derives from its accepted opposition to commercialism" (9). In the debates about legalizing surrogacy contracts in the United States and the UK, for instance, opponents have argued that such contracts attach a price tag to the priceless—children and childbearing. This is closely connected to the idea of "pure" versus "wicked" surrogacy, whereby the "pure" surrogate creates a child out of maternal love, while the "wicked" one "prostitutes her maternity" (Cannell 1990, 683). Surrogates' consistent devaluation of the surrogacy fee in effect fulfills two functions: it confirms the conviction that children cannot be bought or sold and simultaneously establishes the motivation of the surrogate as "pure"—providing an invaluable "gift."

Apart from these cultural beliefs and metaphors, the emphasis on "surrogates as angels" is possibly influenced by the actual working of commercial surrogacy in the United States, where some agencies are known to have refused to accept candidates who indicated that the surrogacy fee was their primary motivation (Ragone 1994). To downplay the pecuniary image of surrogacy, agencies instead encourage their surrogates to think of themselves as "true angels" who "make dreams come true" (Anleu 1992; Ragone 1994). In reproductive contexts in the United States, such idioms can be connected with Christianity and the scriptures of the New Testament, which refers to gifts of "eternal life" and the "child as gift" (Layne 1999). But are these idioms of divinity and gift giving evoked in countries where agencies have different structures and in cultures where Christianity has less of an influence?

In her ethnography of Israeli surrogacy, Teman (2010) discovered that surrogates in Israel more readily accept their motivations as primarily economic, but they too develop a gift rhetoric during the process of surrogacy. Teman calls this "the power of the surrogate-intended mother intimacy to shape the contractual relationship into a gift relationship" (209). Unlike in the United States, the child is not the primary gift that the Israeli surrogate gives; instead, she sees herself as giving another woman, with whom she has developed a close friendship or a familial, sisterly bond, the priceless gift of motherhood. The surrogates in Teman's study may have accepted their pecuniary motives more readily than their counterparts in the United States do, but they were as vocal about establishing their angelic nature. For instance, by equating surrogacy with a *mitzvah* (a good deed that Jews are obligated to perform before God), surrogates in Teman's study saw themselves as "positioned directly under God." One of Teman's respondents captured the narrative perfectly when she described herself as "once an angel, always an angel" (296). Teman also reports other metaphors appropriated by the surrogates to emphasize their true motivation for engaging in surrogacy. For instance, surrogates in Teman's study routinely described surrogacy not just as a "sacred" but also as a "heroic quest," where surrogates as heroes are expected to overcome a series of "hurdles" (245). Alternatively, they imagined themselves to be on a "mission"—to make a family and to make an intended mother a real mother (264).

As one might expect, participants in surrogacy in different parts of the world draw on disparate cultural idioms to make sense of the process. Indeed, why would actors in India, the United States, and Israel use similar idioms for meaning-making? But curiously, idioms do cross borders, and motivations for choosing surrogacy are very often couched in the language of the divine. Given the outright commercial nature of surrogacy in India, one could speculate that Indian surrogates would emphasize their angelic nature and their power to give and serve as messengers of God, much like surrogates in the rest of the world. In the next part of the discussion, though, I demonstrate that while the familiar "gift," "God's labor," and "mission" metaphors are evoked within the process of surrogacy in India, they are used in unexpected ways. In fact, the metaphor of gift giving is almost absent from the narratives of the Indian surrogates themselves. In her work on surrogates in a clinic in India, Kalindi Vora (2010) found that while some surrogates did mention their "power to give," they simultaneously emphasized the important role of the doctors in facilitating this ability to "give" and provide something that is "usually in the domain of a godly gift" (4). While surrogates in Vora's study used the rhetoric of "giving," albeit cautiously, surrogates in my study did not perceive themselves as gift givers at all. The angelic gift-giving surrogate of the Euro-American and Israeli contexts transforms into a needy gift receiver in India, blessed by different avatars of the divine. The idioms of "mission" and "angel," in turn, are evoked by the new messengers of God, the other women involved in surrogacy—doctors, brokers, and intended mothers.

FROM ANGELIC GIFT GIVERS TO NEEDY GIFT RECEIVERS

Why do the narratives manifest so differently in the Indian context? Why do Indian surrogates not portray themselves as angels giving the "true gift of life" to the intended parents? It is likely that differences based on class, race, and nation between the gift giver (surrogate) and the gift receiver (intended parents) make the narrative less credible. How can a desperately poor woman from a village in India possibly be giving a gift to an upper-class Caucasian couple from Los Angeles? Sayantani DasGupta and Shamita Das Dasgupta (2010) provide another explanation—whether it be in organ donation or in surrogacy, the rhetoric of "gift of life" has little cultural resonance in South Asian societies, which "value relationships over autonomy, interdependence over self-governance and group identity over individualism" (140). In her work on philanthropy and humanitarianism in New Delhi, Erica Bornstein (2012) provides an ethnographic account of instances where the language of "gift giving" may not translate across cultures. Bornstein finds that in India, Maussian assumptions of the reciprocal nature of giving are challenged in many instances where "those who give strive to release themselves from any future contract" (14). She connects this to the valorization of anonymous gift giving within Hinduism, with the motivation being tied to the ultimate form of renunciation. Much as gifts to strangers have different interpretations across cultures, gifts to family translate differently as well. Gifts to family are considered a social obligation.

While Vedic scriptures and cultural codes may well contribute to the different construction of gift giving by surrogates, another, more immediate factor is the disciplinary project at the clinic and hostels. As discussed in chapter 4, in the formal and informal counseling sessions, hostel matron Divya explicitly constructs surrogacy as God's gift to needy mothers and coaches surrogates to treat surrogacy not as a business but as a divine gift. The underlying instruction is to be virtuous, not greedy or business-minded, and to never negotiate the payment. Daksha is a 20-year-old surrogate and the mother of three children. I meet her on the day her surrogate pregnancy is confirmed. Daksha knows that just one surrogate birth will not give her enough money, but she echoes Divya's instructions: "I will use the money to educate my children and repair my house. I know I won't have anything left for later, but I don't want to do it [surrogacy] again. Matron Madam is right. God has been generous this time. *He has given me the biggest gift* [emphasis added]—the opportunity to help my family. I don't want to be greedy and try for the second time."

Gauri, another surrogate mother, thinks of this opportunity as God's gift to a needy mother, and like Daksha, she does not want to be greedy: "I pray to Sai Baba [a spiritual guru]—I have a lot of faith in him. *I know this is his gift to a poor mother* [emphasis added]. I don't think I'll go for this again. I don't want to be greedy."

The gift metaphor as used by the Indian surrogates has a powerful corollary—it converts the picture of the angelic gift giver, often associated with surrogates elsewhere, to that of a needy gift receiver. While surrogates in other places are "angels" and "missionaries," choosing to give a gift to the intended parents, God makes the choices for Indian surrogates. The missionary zeal and the idiom of "divine gift giving," however, are not entirely absent in India. They are aggressively evoked by three different sets of actors—the doctor, the brokers, and the intended mothers.

"I AM GRATEFUL THAT I CAN BE A PART OF THIS DIVINE INTERVENTION": THE DOCTOR AND HER "MISSION"

In my first conversation with Dr. Khanderia, she talks about her profession and what motivates her: "Just a few days ago a woman came volunteering to be a surrogate. She brought her two-year-old child with her. I told her that to start the treatment she would need to stop breastfeeding. She told me that unless I can pay her for buying some milk she cannot stop breastfeeding her child! She didn't have enough money to buy even a bottle of milk. That is the state of the women here."

Dr. Khaderia thinks of her involvement in surrogacy as nothing less than a mission. She is, in her own words, a missionary, not very different from Mother Teresa. "I am giving a woman, who cannot have a baby of her own, a baby. And I am giving a woman, who will do anything to feed her starving child, money that is enough to not just feed the child but also send it to school, build a house, become independent. I am very influenced by Mother Teresa. This is my mission and I am grateful that I can be a part of this divine intervention to change two sets of lives."

Dr. Khanderia's construction of assisted conception as "divine" is not unusual. Scholars of infertility, for instance, have recorded that such recourse to divinity enables doctors and patients to make sense of issues such as the success and failure of assisted reproductive techniques (Bharadwaj 2000; Inhorn 2011). Doctors actively counsel clients to accept the limits of what can be achieved through science and medicine, beyond which the work of God becomes involved. But just as interesting is the doctor's construction of her role within the divine intervention as a mission inspired by Mother Teresa. To reiterate her missionary nature, Dr. Khanderia expands on all the services she provides to the surrogates, often unrelated to her clinical responsibilities: "My job is the infertility treatment. Of course I get paid for that, whatever extra care I give to surrogates or the couple I do free of cost. . . . I am sure no doctor in the U.S. would bother about all this. But I go to the extent of making sure the surrogate has a bank account and all the money goes into that account and not her husband's."

On the one hand, most of the doctor's claims are true. She plays an active role in the negotiation of wages for the surrogates, in setting up bank accounts, and even in the assignment of intended parents to surrogates. While the ultimate "match" is determined by the medical compatibility between surrogate and intended mother, Dr. Khanderia has an unofficial policy of assigning the highest-paying couples to the surrogates who she believes have the most urgent needs. On the other hand, it cannot be denied that the doctor makes enormous profits and publicity from this international business in wombs. During my entire fieldwork experience, spanning more than six years, Dr. Khanderia did not once divulge how much profit she makes per surrogacy arrangement. Moreover, despite her self-proclaimed missionary nature and claims of egalitarianism, the system of recruitment, the formal and informal brokers, and the surveillance techniques used in the hostels are not only discriminatory but also potentially exploitative. In all her conversations, Dr. Khanderia manages to circumvent these exploitative instances by claiming little involvement in either the brokerage system or the hostels: "These are all initiatives of enterprising women. I do not support the brokers, financially or otherwise."

The brokers, however, have a different version to tell.

"HE HAS COME IN MY DREAMS AND ADVISED ME": BROKER VIMLA IN "GOD'S SERVICE"

I meet Vimla for the first time in the clinic's courtyard. She has brought two new women to the clinic. She met these women at a neighboring village and persuaded them to try surrogacy. Vimla rides a scooter (which she uses to transport the women to the clinic), is better dressed than most of the nurses, carries an expensive-looking leather purse, and wears several gold bangles—all of which are indicators of her relative affluence. She is followed closely by her entourage of surrogates and egg donors, women that she has brought to the clinic. Some want a ride back to their village, and others just clutch onto her as the only familiar face in the city. Vimla starts talking about her role in the surrogacy process:

> I am the eldest in my family and I need to take care of everyone. If I had become a surrogate myself, I would have to lie in bed for nine months. So I thought of an alternative. I asked Doctor Madam if she wants me to get her some surrogates and Madam agreed. I started getting patients from the hospital where I work as a midwife. Everyone in the clinic, the staff and the Doctor respect me. I have a good relationship with them. Well, I do get them a lot of surrogates. Almost every day I get them surrogates and egg donors. They respect me here.

Although Vimla believes that the medical staff at the clinic respect her, most nurses joke about her and refer to her as the "greedy broker." The doctor refuses to even acknowledge Vimla's role in the surrogacy process and emphasizes that Vimla is not hired or "paid a cut" by the clinic. Vimla, however, tells the story differently. She not only emphasizes that the doctor pays her a fee, but she also complains that this fee structure is very unfair.

> Doctor Madam pays me a cut. Earlier my cut was proportional to the amount the couple agreed to pay for the surrogate. So if a surrogate got Rs. 1 lakh [$2,000], I got Rs. 5,000 [$100]. If she got Rs. 2 lakhs, I got Rs. 10,000. But now my cut has been fixed. The surrogates also pay me just a fixed amount, Rs. 10,000 [$200], irrespective of whether the party pays the surrogate 1 lakh or 4 lakhs. My share never increases. Of course, I would prefer to get a percentage of the total amount paid to the surrogate. But what can I do, I have to agree to whatever they give.

Ironically, right after presenting her grudges about unfair payment, Vimla explains why she continues in her role despite the unfair pay—the money is secondary for her. She is a broker to fulfill a divine mission, and listen to the voice of God.

> I am a bhakt [devotee] of Sai Baba [a Hindu sage]. Since I started this, he has come in my dreams and advised me. He has told me, "Vimla, you cannot

leave this, whatever happens." Sometimes I get frustrated that I feel like leaving all this but then I think of these poor women [the women from the villages] and tell myself I have to continue for their sake. For them I am like an elder sister, savior, mentor, all rolled into one. This is what makes me happy. I know the money is bad, but this thing has become my way of doing God's service now.

While Vimla claims that she continues her "service" merely for the welfare of the surrogates, all the surrogates complain about the amount of the brokerage fee Vimla charges, especially since the only service she provides is to introduce them to the clinic. Although Vimla claims that she takes the $200 after delivery, several surrogates mention that Vimla insists on getting paid as soon as they get their first installment of payment after three months of confirmed pregnancy. While the nurses have labeled her the "greedy one," the surrogates refer to her as the "crocodile" eating up their savings (see chapter 8). Vimla claims she is unaffected by these "misunderstandings": "I did not come here to make friends with anyone. I am a believer. I pray, I follow God's orders. Their bad names for me cannot hurt me. We are all misunderstood. That's the irony of doing God's work, you cannot beat your own drum [*dheendhora peetna*]. But I know, none of them [the clinic and the surrogates] can make it without me."

Undeterred by all the criticism, Vimla is planning to expand her "service" and start a surrogacy hostel. During the course of my fieldwork, she managed to persuade the doctor to pay the initial start-up costs for her hostel. In 2011, "missionary" Vimla had become not just a surrogacy broker but also a hostel matron.

"I HAVE SPENT MY ENTIRE LIFE FOLLOWING GOD'S ORDERS": BROKER KANTA AND HER "GOD'S WORK"

Kanta is a nurse, midwife, and surrogacy broker but prefers to call herself either a social worker or God's worker. She states that she has a long-standing relationship with both God and Dr. Khanderia. Before the advent of surrogacy, Kanta brought women with complicated pregnancies from her village to the clinic. She also persuaded married women with children in her village to get sterilization operations or use other forms of [long-term] contraception. As part of her "service," she would take the women to the city to get surgery/contraceptives. Kanta insists that she doesn't charge any fee for the services rendered—from either the client or the doctor. Now she spends most of her time persuading women in her village to become surrogates and brings them to the clinic.

I visit Kanta in her new apartment in a village near Garv. The apartment is still under construction and is being financed entirely by the money her daughter-in-law got from delivering twins for an Indian couple settled in the United States. Kanta talks about her yearning to be in God's service. "My husband and I are very religious people. Lord Krishna has guided us in everything we do, whether it be my nurse work or this. He teaches me the right from the wrong. Ask anyone in my village and they know Kanta. There is no household here that has not been helped by me, in some way or the other. I have spent my entire life following God's orders. *Jai Shree Krishna* [Lord Krishna be praised]."

Kanta emphasizes that the business aspect of surrogacy is not significant. She works as a broker for the "blessings" she gets for her good deeds—blessings from the couple, from the surrogates, and from God. "For me the money is not that important. It's about the service. Money comes and goes but the blessings of the couple who hire surrogates and the surrogates, who need the money, will be there for us. You see this house that I am building now, it's like God is blessing me for all my good deeds."

Unlike Vimla, Kanta continues her "service" from the sidelines. Her business dealings are somewhat different from Vimla's aggressive brokering and she is not talked about much at the clinic. Kanta charges her cut only when a pregnancy is successful. The amount the brokers charge is important in delineating each step of the surrogacy process, but just as instructive are the determined efforts made by the brokers to construct their business as a "mission" and downplay the pecuniary nature of their role.

Once a woman has been recruited by such self-proclaimed missionaries, the next step in the induction program is a meeting with the surrogate counselor, Divya. Much like the doctors and brokers, hostel matron Divya has her own divine version of surrogacy and her role in it.

"I KNEW GOD HAD OTHER PLANS FOR ME. MY MISSION IS TO SPREAD SMILES": SURROGACY COUNSELOR AND HOSTEL MATRON DIVYA

Divya was in the seventh month of pregnancy, surrogate for a couple from the United States, when I met her in 2006. Divya and her husband worked as bank tellers in a city. The bank job paid them "enough to survive," but not enough for their elder son's surgery. I met Divya again when I revisited the field the following year. Even during my first visit Divya seemed exceptional—she was the only surrogate from outside the state and the only one with a college education. But when I met her the following year, it was impossible to compare her to other financially desperate surrogates. Divya seemed to have done very well for herself. Dr. Khanderia, realizing the advantages of hiring a former surrogate as a counselor for potential surrogates, offered her the job of a counselor at the clinic.

Divya recalls her day of "calling," which motivated her to take up the job. "Once I had delivered the baby to Anne, I was ready to return to my hometown. But suddenly it struck me: 'What has just happened is big, it is huge!' You have made an American couple smile forever. You have given your family a new life. And you will just leave this and go back to ordinary life again? I knew I had a bigger purpose in life. I knew God had other plans for me. I had to listen to him."

Divya thinks of her new job as not just a "calling" but also her good *karma*. "Maybe it's *karma*, do a good thing and get real returns. My son did not need his surgery eventually. That was God's plan for us, and so is this. You know how much I get paid here as a counselor? You won't be able to guess! Rs 35,000 [$700] every month, can you imagine that! That is three times the salary I got as a bank teller."

Apart from being a counselor and mediator, in her final avatar Divya is the owner-matron of the first surrogacy hostel in that region. The hostel is financed partly by the clinic and partly by the monthly maintenance fees paid by intended parents. By my second trip to the field, Divya had started adding another floor to her two-story apartment. She and her husband together earned about $1,000 per month, enough to pay for two cooks, two maids, one handyman, and one driver for the hostel/apartment. Divya imitates the strategy of her mentor, Dr. Khanderia, in not revealing how much profit she makes out of this establishment. But the "fruits" of her karma are visible in her residence.

I sit with Divya as she watches her nanny bathe her infant son in the newly refurbished Jacuzzi zone in her apartment. She describes the initial reason for starting the hostel: "When I moved to Garv last year I realized that a lot of the surrogates traveling from far were not getting enough rest. There was a surrogate who was planning to be a surrogate for Anne's next baby and I could see that she is not getting enough rest. Anne and I share a very special relationship ever since I delivered a son for her. I started the hostel basically for Anne, to make sure she gets the best deal possible. Of course now Doctor Madam sends many surrogates here."

Although Divya started the hostel as homage to the intended parents, she believes her mission has expanded to "spreading smiles" to all the actors involved in surrogacy:

> This hostel has expanded like anything in its first year. But I am not running this hostel for business. I do all this because I know what a struggle it is for the surrogates—in a new place, away from family, in hiding. I have been blessed by God once. I want to be able to share the fruits of that with these poor women. *My mission is to spread smiles*, make sure Doctor Madam is happy, the American couples are happy and the surrogates are well cared for. I hardly get any time with my family because of all these responsibilities, but it feels good at the end of the day.

Like her mentor and employer, Divya interprets her role in the surrogacy industry as a divine intervention and partly a selfless mission to "spread smiles." It is not that surprising that program managers and brokers downplay the pecuniary nature of their involvement in the business of wombs by emphasizing their missionary zeal and their role as God's messengers. Far more startling is a similar missionary narrative evoked by another set of women involved in the surrogacy process—the intended mothers.

"THIS FEELS LIKE A WORTHY CAUSE": INTENDED MOTHERS TALK

Oprah Winfrey opened her show on infertility in October 2007 by promising to reveal "why childless couples will stop at *nothing* to have a baby" and asked her viewers in an ominous voice-over, "How far would you go?" The answer for one couple, Jennifer and Kendall, was "India." Her reporter, Oprah promised, would travel to a clinic in India to figure out why some North American couples are choosing a developing country like India to try and have a child of their own. At the end of the show Oprah concluded that couples like Jennifer and Kendall are no less than brave missionaries to countries that few would ever dream of visiting. Many of the transnational clients I met at Garv emphasized this "mission" as their primary motivation in choosing a clinic in India.

Anne is an intended mother from the United States and has hired two surrogates in two years. Anne assures me that her decision to come to

India was not based on financial considerations: "It's not because of the cost difference. I already spent a lot at home. People travel to the U.S. to get a surrogate and here I am traveling out of it into someplace as far as India. My friends think I am very brave to be traveling to this country. I mean if you take one look at the streets outside, you would know why. But we decided on India because we thought women here would be more conservative—drug- and alcohol-free."

While Anne recognizes the advantages of hiring a presumably drug-free, conservative woman, she also emphasizes the "bravery" of her decision. Much like the missionaries of the past ventured into dangerous zones to spread the message of Christ and rescue the "natives," Anne is venturing into the streets of Garv so as to change the life of a miserable Indian woman. "What makes me happy about my decision is that the [life] of my surrogate would change with the money. Without our help her family would not be able to get out of the situation they are in, not even in a million years."

The desire to contribute to a worthy cause was echoed by several of my international respondents. Judy, another intended mother from the United States, gives a similar justification:

> I have tried IVF five times in Florida and already spent a packet. Money is not an issue with us since we are both physicians. The big attraction was that surrogates are easily available, willing and well taken care of. Also, in the U.S. we have no control over the surrogates—after the contract is signed they may even become inaccessible, may do drugs, whatever, who knows . . . Most importantly we realized that for surrogates here the amount we pay would be a life-altering one while in the U.S. it's just some extra money. What really helped us take this decision was that we knew our surrogate wouldn't spend the money for drugs or a flat-screen TV. She would be using it to feed her family, build her own house. It would feel good to make such a change in someone's life. I am not religious, but this seemed almost like God's work, call it a worthy cause . . . a mission.

Eve, an intended mother from Canada, reveals her primary reason for abandoning her search for commercial surrogates in California: "It was not just the cost thing. I was looking for an Indian surrogate because in the U.S., with women . . . you know with the ones who would want to do this for money, you never know—they could be smoking, drinking, doing drugs. An Indian lady is very unlikely to have such vices. And at the end of it all, it boils down to having a healthy surrogate. . . . And tell me, what's wrong in coming down here? Why question my intentions to help a whole family out of their crazy situation?"

What is intriguing is that Anne, Judy, and Eve construct the Indian surrogate not only as desperately poor, but also as "worthy" poor. Unlike surrogates in the United States, who allegedly would use the money for drugs and other frivolous consumption, Indian surrogates are expected to use the money productively. In her interactions with an American commissioning couple planning to hire a surrogate in India, sociologist Arlie Hochschild found that the couple saw their relationship with the surrogate as a "mutually beneficial one"—much like "paying a stranger to provide a professionally supervised service" (2012, 83). Curiously, none of the transnational clients I interacted with over the five years described their relationship with the surrogate in such explicitly market terms. While most clients were willing to acknowledge the range of benefits of hiring a surrogate in India, from easy laws to control over the surrogates, they reiterated that these benefits were secondary. Their primary motivation, the clients insisted, was to transform the life of a family living in desperate poverty. Hiring a surrogate from a distant Third World nation was visualized as another form of development aid, with the hiring couple playing the role of brave missionaries battling all odds to help the needy.[4]

Scholarship on transnational adoption has indicated that adopting parents often evoke similar narratives, in which the desire to adopt children is constructed as a form of international aid (Briggs 2003; Cartwright 2005; Volkman 2005). Ideologies of rescue, care, and compassion are rampant in accounts given by people involved in transnational adoptions. Curiously, even in the absence of the "abandoned child in need of being rescued," transnational clients of reproductive services seem to give similar accounts of "moral adoption." For many transnational clients of surrogacy, the overwhelming narrative is reminiscent of a missionary zeal. Another narrative frequently used, especially by clients from the Indian diaspora, was that of their "excessive generosity." Intended mothers often emphasized their generosity and spoke of all the payments made in cash and kind, payments not required by either the clinic or the contract. Preeti, from New Jersey, is an American citizen, but her parents are Indian.

She talks about her decision to gift a piece of land to the surrogate, but emphasizes that it is not "charity":

> I am a doctor myself and I have really been busy the last few months. I did call my surrogate every day in the beginning, and then it became a weekly or fortnightly call. But I won't forget her after the delivery. We plan to send her gifts every year on my child's birthday. . . . I want to buy her a piece of land on top of all the cash. I know my husband thinks I am being silly, but I want to do it for her. I won't call it charity. She has given me a lot. But we have given her a lot as well. This should get her life all set.

Kavya, an Indian settled in South Africa, mentions her husband's generosity toward the surrogate and her family. Unlike Preeti, Kavya compares this generosity to her other "charity" work back home:

> I went and visited my surrogate at her hut in the village. She really has a hard life. I feel for her. All those kids, and such a useless husband. I did not know what to do to help her so my husband took control. He has decided to gift her husband a motorcycle; maybe that will make him more enterprising! We are also planning to help out with the education of her eldest child. We will do as much as we can. We donate quite regularly to community-run schools back home as well. This is even better—I feel so much closer to this family.

Although intended parents from the Indian diaspora were less direct about their "mission" than their counterparts with no Indian connection, the parallels between payment for surrogacy and donation crept into many of the narratives. By critically appraising the narratives of the intended mothers, I am not aiming to question or doubt their actual generosity or intention. It might well be that these extra payments allow the surrogates to temporarily better their lives. I discuss the longer-run impacts of surrogacy, and the material benefits for the surrogates, in the epilogue of this book. Interestingly, the "mission" and "charity" narrative and the construction of payment as donation to the needy fit perfectly with the disciplining project described in chapter 4. In spite of the various advantages for the clients hiring surrogates at Garv, the rates can remain the lowest in the world partly because the women are framed not as workers with desirable skills or qualities but as desperate and needy mothers. The picture of a needy woman legitimizes the low pay, and the framing of this transaction as a "worthy cause" equates the payment to a donation—informal and/or voluntary. The surrogate, by being "trained" to be a virtuous and nurturing mother and simultaneously a professional and docile worker, would hesitate to engage in negotiating the wages she gets from this labor. After all, this work is God's gift to her and she is to do this work not out of greed but to fulfill her familial responsibilities. And after all, she is just another womb waiting in line to be rescued by a noble foreigner.

6 ✒ EMBODIED LABOR AND NEO-EUGENICS

My sister and I have been in this business for a while. When Doctor Madam started egg donation at this clinic, my sister was the first one to give her eggs and I was the next. Madam gave me Rs.1000 [$20] for that. I've given my eggs ten times since then. It's a very painful procedure. But it pays for my family's monthly expenses so I do it. . . . Then last year (as a surrogate) I delivered a baby girl to a couple from the U.S. They liked me so they have hired me again, for their second baby. But I won't give any more eggs. I am tired. I need to give this body a rest. After all it's my body that is paying the monthly bills.

—Rita, surrogate mother for a couple from the United States, 2007

SURROGACY AS EMBODIED LABOR

We cannot possibly discuss surrogacy without talking about the body. In essence, a surrogate is using her body, specifically her womb and her uterus, to earn income. In addition, gestational surrogacy, by separating the reproducer's body or womb from her genetic material, ensures that the only requirements clients and doctors emphasize are corporal in nature: a healthy womb that produces a healthy baby. Unlike in traditional surrogacy, in gestational surrogacy the surrogate's genetic makeup becomes irrelevant. It is no surprise, then, that the surrogate's body is both appraised and monitored at each stage of the surrogacy process—at recruitment and throughout the disciplinary regimen at the hostel. But the body is not just subjected to a course of discipline; it is just as much a space of resistance for the surrogates and a place for them to claim a sense of control.

A close examination of the role of the body in this new form of labor first warrants a review of the way the worker's body has been previously discussed in the literature on the sociology of work. Bodies are not new to studies of work, but somehow they remain in the margins (Wolkowitz 2006). This marginality of the body from the sociology of work can be partly attributed to the fact that marginalized populations have historically provided most of the work that directly involves the body. Servants, slaves, and women have performed these types of work, largely without pay. Not surprisingly, such work is often labeled "reproductive" or dismissed as existing outside the labor market. While sociologists of work have paid relatively little attention to bodies, classic texts in the sociology of the body (Burkitt 1999; Shilling 1993; Turner 1984), as well as feminist scholarship (Brook 1999; Grosz 1994; Jaggar and Bordo 1989; Weitz 2003), show curiously little interest in experiences of embodiment in paid work (Wolkowitz 2006). The bridge between bodies and labor remained a relatively unexplored territory.

The past few decades have witnessed what sociologist Miliann Kang has called a turn toward "bringing bodies back in" in sociology and feminist scholarship (Kang 2003, 821). However, with postmodernism, attention often moves away from an engagement with action and practice toward more philosophical conceptualizations of the body.[1] Curiously, in the postmodern world, even the term "body work" has little to do with the corporality of paid and unpaid work. It tends to refer to techniques of the self, including dieting or consumption of services, like cosmetic surgery (Black 2004; Gimlin 2002) and is rarely used to refer to work performed by paid workers. Perhaps that is why Kang (2003) in her work on nail salons chooses the term "body labor" to describe the provision of body-related services and the management of the feelings that accompany it. Some other examples of such body labor, or provision of body-related services, that speak to the intersection of gender, body, and paid work are sex work, nursing, and professional massage (George 2000; Oerton and Phoenix 2001; Twigg 2000). The concepts highlighted by scholars writing on body labor are the combined expectations of emotional labor and sexualized performances from the worker (Wolkowitz 2006, 77).[2] These professions usually involve women working on the bodies of their (often male) clients. The other commonality is the high level of touch engaged in primarily for monetary gain.

The lens of body labor, however, cannot fully capture the extreme corporality of surrogacy as paid labor. Surrogacy, like salon work, sex work, and nursing, does involve body-related services. But instead of servicing the clients' bodies, the surrogates are deploying their own bodies to deliver the ultimate product. The involvement of the body in surrogacy is different from its use in most other kinds of labor where the employer has no intrinsic interest in the body of the worker. It can be argued that employers of (women) workers in customer service and "aesthetic labor" like fashion retail also give great importance to embodied dispositions (sexual desirability, deportment, dressing style) of their workers (Witz, Warhurst, and Nickson 2003). But there are profound differences in expectations about embodied dispositions of workers in service industries and the kind of worker embodiment required in surrogacy. Surrogacy is an extreme example of the manifestation of worker embodiment, where body is the ultimate site of labor, where the resources, the skills, and the ultimate product are derived primarily from the body of the laborer. The worker's embodiment is essentially *living* in the commodity produced—literally in the form of the worker's bodily fluids, her blood and sweat.

Given the limitations of both the "body labor" lens and the "aesthetic labor" lens in capturing the corporality of surrogacy as labor, I use the term "embodied labor" to capture the uniqueness of surrogacy as a labor process. Embodied labor such as commercial surrogacy in India (and to some extent sex work or wet nursing) in effect involves a rental of the use of one's body by somebody else, in which the body of the worker is the fundamental and ultimate site, resource, requirement, and (arguably) product. The necessary requirements to be a commercial surrogate pertain almost exclusively to the surrogate's body: she should be under the age of 40 with at least one healthy child, should not be breast-feeding her own child, should not have had more than three pregnancies, should have no history of miscarriage, should have a healthy uterus and be disease-free. The corporality of the surrogate's work and the centrality of her body are written into the surrogacy contract itself in the form of her agreement to refrain from the use of alcohol and cigarettes, her willingness to refrain from sexual contact with her husband and to stop her regular work (including housework) for the entire period of treatment and pregnancy. In addition, the surrogacy contract requires repeated invasive techniques: the surrogate has to be willing to receive daily injections, undergo periodic blood tests, and ingest all medicines and vitamins vital for fetal growth. She must also agree to abort the fetus or undergo selective reduction, caesarean section, or intrauterine fetal surgery, according to the doctor's recommendation.

In this chapter, however, I use the term "embodied labor" not just to highlight the critical corporal nature of this work but to analyze the surrogate's response to the disciplinary project outlined in chapter 4—the clinic's attempt to produce the perfect "mother-worker" body, whether at the clinic or at the surrogacy hostels. As the hyper-medicalized body of the surrogate comes under increased scrutiny, the surrogate not only retains control over her body but often *reclaims* control by using her body for labor. To do this, the surrogate negotiates with not just the clinic but also her family, especially her husband and in-laws. The multiple arenas of resistances and negotiations by the surrogate in turn reveal the many layers of domination, at the level of the family, the clinic, and the state.

It is important to keep the distinct nature of biomedicalization in India and the historical context of the Indian postcolonial state, outlined in chapter 2 of this book, in mind in order to understand the surrogates' negotiations and resistances as laborers. Just as the development of modern birth is not uniform across countries, forms of negotiation and resistance at the micro-political level are also distinct. The surrogates are responding to unprecedented levels of medicalization in a country with a relatively low rate of biomedicalization and professionalization of childbirth. But their negotiations and resistances are also shaped by the anti-natalist state agenda and the historically high level of state surveillance of the fertility of lower-class women. I identify four types of everyday negotiations by the women involved in this embodied form of labor: (1) portrayal of surrogacy as "productive," (2) (re)negotiation of birth-control decisions to participate in this form of labor, (3) resistance to the "scissor" (caesarean section), and finally (4) negotiating the nature of prenatal and postnatal care. Although these negotiations are at the micro-political level—with their families (husbands and in-laws) and with the clinic, this chapter illustrates how they are affected by and have repercussions at the macro level.

"MY BODY PAYS THE BILLS": SURROGACY AS PRODUCTIVE MOTHERHOOD

One of the key features of the Indian state's population control program has been the focus on the responsible woman who desires and plans for a small family. National and state-level propaganda use a variety of communication methods and media—illustrated pamphlets, puppet shows, radio and television advertisements, and more—to promote its official slogan *"chhota parivar, sukhi parivar"* (a small family is a happy family) (Chatterjee and Riley 2001; Conly and Camp 1992; Dharmalingam 1995). The official intention of much of this propaganda is to "empower women" to make family planning decisions "by instructing them on the appropriate merits and methods of contraception" (Chatterjee and Riley 2001, 834). For instance, a recent family planning video uses the latest government slogan, *"pati patni kare vichar, swastha naari swastha parivar"* (husband wife plan together, a healthy woman means a healthy family), which ostensibly campaigns for joint decisions. But despite the slogan, the videos and images hold the woman responsible for either using long-term contraceptives like Copper-T IUD or persuading her husband to use a condom. In rural areas, older family planning posters analyzed by anthropologists Nilanjana Chatterjee and Nancy Riley (2001) over a decade ago are still in vogue, and are still visible on the walls of stores and in rail and bus stations.[3] For instance, a poster targeting women specifically shows a sari-clad woman with a small boy and the caption "Before you have another child, think." Such constructions of women as "primary agents of change" disregard the extent of male (and familial) control over female sexuality and reproductive decisions (Chatterjee and Riley 2001, 834).

In all its forms, the anti-natalist propaganda of the Indian state portrays the fertile bodies of lower-class women as recklessly reproductive and to be blamed for the women's poverty. The narratives of surrogates reveal this state propaganda. Varsha is a 38-year-old mother of three children and is a surrogate for a couple from North India. She recalls the many visits by the *dai* (family planning nurse):[4]

> I never used any contraceptive, just regulated intercourse according to my monthly cycle. But the *dai* [woman from the family planning clinic] would stop at our hut on her visits and tell me to think of getting the operation [sterilization or long-term implants]. "But why do you not get it?" she would say. She showed my sister and me pictures of women with one daughter, where the daughter and the mother would be smiling. She sometimes scolded us and said, "That is why your condition is like this. The more babies you have, the poorer you get, do you not understand that?" Perhaps she is right. If I had not had my last child, the first two would be happier. *But now the tables have turned* [emphasis added]. You see,

it is my fourth pregnancy [the surrogate birth] that will make my entire family happy.

For Varsha, "the tables have turned" with her participation in the embodied labor of surrogacy. The state portrayal of her reckless fertility as an obstruction to her family's prosperity is challenged by her "productive motherhood." Her surrogate pregnancy will, in fact, enable her family to better their financial situation and get out of poverty. Commercial surrogacy drives women to think of their bodies as a possible source of value, a value denied by the state itself. Although only a third of the women in this study identify as housewives, most others work in informal or contract work with low, irregular incomes. The money earned through surrogacy often becomes a source of pride, and an indicator of their productivity.

Rita is a 29-year-old surrogate for a non-resident Indian (NRI) couple from the United States. Rita talks about the "family business" of engaging in this embodied labor:

This hospital is almost like my house now. I've come here so often. My mother is a *dai*, she knows Doctor Madam for many years now. She often brings women with complicated pregnancies to this clinic. My sisters and my sister-in-law have also been surrogates. I am the fourth to be a surrogate in my family. Our whole family runs on this! I've already delivered a baby girl to a couple last year and they asked me to do it again this year. I used the money to pay back some debt and reconstruct the roof of my house. I put the rest of it in the bank in a fixed deposit. My husband and I have a joint account. He is a good husband. He wants me to make the decisions about this money. This is the first time I am working out of the house and am earning so much—much more than he ever has. He was reluctant, but he let me do this the second time. I want to buy a house with the money I earn this time.

Rita is one of the few to emphasize the irony of surrogacy in an otherwise anti-natalist state. Later in the conversation she reiterates Varsha's claim, "the tables have turned," and reflects on the changing role played by her mother, Kanta, an informal surrogacy broker introduced in chapter 5: "My mother used to convince women in her village to get sterilization operations or use other forms of [long-term] contraceptives.

She would take poor women from our village to the city to get surgeries. But now with surrogacy catching up, she spends more time bringing surrogates to Madam's clinic. Now things are different. Mothers of our age can make good use of our bodies and our motherhood. We can make good money by having babies."

Surrogacy thus converts the "wasteful" reproducing bodies of lower-class women into productive ones. Surrogates often stress the productive uses of the money earned through surrogacy. They emphasize that the money would be invested in bringing about change—making a difference in the lives of their families—and would not be spent on daily expenses.

Puja is a 27-year-old surrogate who had already delivered a baby for an Indian couple and was pregnant for the second time in two years. She talks about spending the money earned from surrogacy:

> My husband feels proud that I have earned so much money and done something that even he couldn't have. Well, he should—look at how much the money I earned has changed our lives. I built one house and bought another plot of land in the city with the money I got from my first surrogacy. When I become a surrogate again, I will build another house on that plot. I want to do this again and again. He [her husband] did not want me to do this again. But I convinced him that we need the money to educate our children. My father-in-law was very against it as well, right from [the] start. But I told him it's my life, I'll do what I feel is right. Right now I am young I have the health, the body and the ability to earn some extra cash, so why shouldn't I?

Puja makes two assertions: First, engaging in surrogacy was her decision and she negotiated this decision with her family. Despite objections by her father-in-law, Puja is able to set her own priorities and become a surrogate. Second, she decides how the money earned through surrogacy will be spent. Both Puja and Rita reiterate that the money earned through surrogacy has brought about life changes. They simultaneously state that their husbands, although reluctant about letting their wives become surrogates, are proud of their wives' accomplishment.

Dipali is a 24-year-old surrogate for a couple from South Africa. A divorcée with three children, Dipali has been living with her brother and his family for more than five years. She wants to use part of the money she earned to buy a piece of land and deposit the rest in a fixed account for her children's education.

When I came here I told Doctor Madam that I am ready for all kinds of treatment—injections, medicines. I just need some strength and God's help. I often bring other women from my community to this clinic. I convince them to try egg donation and then I tell them about surrogacy. I tell them that even if they struggle their entire lifetime they will not be able to earn this much money. Yes, there is a lot of pain in this, but you get results. I ask them to think about it with a clear head and how much they can do for their children with the money.

Dipali compares the pain of surrogacy to the pain of living in an abusive relationship:

I know I have the strength to go through all this for my children. I have suffered the pain and the bleeding. I almost got paralysis twice and had to be hospitalized, because of side effects of some medicines. But I am not complaining about the pain. I worried, I cried, and I complained when my husband used to beat me up in front of my children. That pain is what you do not want. This kind of pain to the body I am willing to take—it will not be wasted—it will give me enough money to make me self-sufficient.

Dipali asserts that she is willing to endure all forms of medical interventions on her body to engage in this labor because she knows it will be productive—it will enable her to become self-sufficient. Sociologist Sharmila Rudrappa (2012) reports similar narratives from the gestational surrogates she interviewed in the Indian city of Bangalore. One of Rudrappa's interviewees, a former garment factory worker, prefers producing a baby to producing garments, as it gives her "the opportunity to be highly productive and creative." The surrogate told Rudrappa, "You wear your shirt a few months and you throw it away. But I make you a baby? You keep that for life. I have made something so much bigger than anything I could ever make in the factory."

Puja, Rita, and Dipali are able to negotiate with their husbands and in-laws and use their bodies to earn money. Their reproductivity, which has historically been framed as a source of their poverty, becomes an indicator of their productivity. They hope to use this money earned to improve their lives and those of their children—by buying a piece of land, building a house, or saving for their children's education and marriage.

SURROGACY, STERILIZATIONS, AND ABORTIONS: (RE)NEGOTIATING BIRTH CONTROL DECISIONS

For the surrogates in the Armaan Maternity Clinic, having control over their reproductive lives and bodies is about being able to use their bodies for paid work and to determine how the money earned is used. Control in this context is also about (re)negotiating birth control decisions with their husbands in order to get involved in surrogacy. Although the everyday negotiations of reproductive decisions are at the local level, they speak to hegemonic discourses that portray the fertility of lower-class women (in the global south) as a drain on the society.

Ramya is a surrogate for a non-resident Indian settled in the United States. She wants to save the money earned and use it for her daughter's marriage. She talks about her decision to become a surrogate:

> I have just one child—a daughter. . . . I got an operation [sterilization] done to prevent further pregnancies. But when I heard about surrogacy I realized that I wanted to do this. I came to the clinic to ask if there was a way to reverse the operation so that I could be a surrogate for someone. I came to the clinic alone. No one in my family knows I am doing this. Even my husband remained reluctant till the end. But I told him *it's my body and I know what I want to do with it* [emphasis added]. Here in the clinic they told me I could be a surrogate even if I have undergone the operation earlier.

Ramya is willing to reverse her sterilization operation in order to engage in the embodied labor of surrogacy. She makes this decision without the knowledge of her family and despite her husband's reluctance. Sterilization (mainly female sterilization) remains the most commonly used method of birth control in India and people often equate the term "family planning" with sterilization (Rutenberg and Landry 1993; Zavier and Padmadas 2000). Government incentives to both users and providers, mentioned in chapter 2, undoubtedly contribute to the predominance of permanent methods, like sterilization, over temporary ones. Most women hear about sterilization from nurses and midwives during the delivery of their own children or from family planning officials visiting their village (Van Hollen 1998, 2003; Ram 2001).[5] In this study, of the 20 surrogates who practiced any form of contraception, 13 were sterilized (see table 2 in appendix B).

Vidya is a 30-year-old surrogate for a couple from Chennai, India. She will use the money to pay for her children's higher education. Vidya has repeatedly been told about sterilization by family planning officers visiting her village but has been postponing the operation.

I have two daughters and one son. My husband wanted one more son, so we decided not to get the operation done. It must have been God's wish that I do this [become a surrogate]. If I had got the operation done, I would have missed this chance to earn money for my children. But now that I am successfully pregnant [as a surrogate mother], I don't think I will try for another son anymore. I know my husband wants a son very badly but I am going to try and convince him. If I have a baby of my own now, I will lose the chance to become a surrogate again. *I want to conserve my body and save my next pregnancy for surrogacy*, in case we need money again [emphasis added]. Doctor Madam does not want surrogates who have more than three babies of their own.

While Ramya contemplates reversing a family planning operation in order to become a surrogate, Vidya wants to "save her next pregnancy" for surrogacy. Vidya has postponed sterilization and resisted the instruction of family planning officials because her husband wanted another son. Now, in order to become a surrogate, she is willing to convince her husband to forgo that son.

Munni, who works as a nanny, is a mother of three children and is a surrogate for an Indian couple settled in the United States. Her husband is unemployed. Munni will use the money from surrogacy to start a street-corner barbershop for her husband.

If I hadn't become a surrogate would I have had more children of my own? No, I don't think so. I already have one too many. The *dai* says to me "If you are so educated, why didn't you get sterilized?" I told her I had the third child because my mother-in-law forced me to. She harassed me every day till I gave her another grandson. She harasses me all the time even though I work outside the house and earn money. When I had my second baby I wanted to get the [sterilization] operation but my husband and mother-in-law didn't let me. So when they said they don't want me to become a surrogate, I said to myself, "Enough. Everyone makes me do things for their own convenience. Have baby, don't have baby, always for your own dreams. This time I will have a baby [as a surrogate] because I want to."

For Munni, using her body for work is a response to the instructions of family planning officials and family members. It becomes a way to assert control over her reproduction and her body. Puja, Rita, Ramya, Vidya, and Munni negotiate with their husbands and in-laws, contemplate reversing family planning operations, and even forgo having their own children in order to become surrogates. They resist the instructions of family planning professionals and the reluctance of family members and ostensibly take control over their bodies by engaging in surrogacy. But while at one level these women appear to fulfill feminist ideals, their life stories are not just heroic tales of resistance. The decisions they make about their own reproduction conform to the global imperative of reducing the fertility of lower-class women in the global south.

Vidya is not the only surrogate to forgo having her own child in order to have a child for someone else. Parvati is 36 and one of the oldest surrogates at the clinic. Her story reveals the multitude of bodily interventions involved in the work of surrogacy.

> When I came here the first time the Doctor said I was too old to donate eggs but I could try for surrogacy. . . . I underwent treatment—injections, vagina check. A lot of extra medication and checkup was necessary because I am older than the rest of the surrogates. During one of the first checkups they realized that I was pregnant with my own child. We have just one child, a boy, and we have always wanted one more. But at that stage, we needed the money more than a baby and I got the baby aborted.

It is more than poignant that Parvati undergoes abortion of her own pregnancy so as to give birth to someone else's child.[6] Later in the conversation, Parvati discloses that she regrets getting the abortion done:

> What I did cannot be reversed now. Maybe it's God's way of punishing me [for the abortion]. . . . Now I am pregnant with triplets and Doctor Madam wants me to go through another abortion [fetal reduction surgery]. I cried so much when Madam told me that. I asked her if I could keep one and they [the intended parents] can keep two. But I know that will not be allowed. My husband consoles me and says, "Once we have enough money, we can have one of our own." But at my age I don't think another one will be possible.

Parvati's story is not unusual. Naseem has been married for more than seven years and is the mother of a three-year-old son. Naseem's decision to become a surrogate is just one event in a web of fertility-related decisions.

> My husband and I had been trying to have a second baby for a while. Everyone asked us why we had stopped at just one and whether I had a problem [conceiving]. I hadn't got the sterilization operation nor were we using any other contraception. When I got pregnant with our second child, he [her husband] was very happy; "now these people can stop asking us questions." But later that month he got laid off from his factory work. He sent me with my sister-in-law to this clinic to get an abortion. There the sister [nurse] told me to get either an operation [sterilization] or IUD insertion. She also told me about surrogacy. I got the abortion and after six months started treatment for this surrogacy. It will be easy to explain to the neighbors when the pregnancy starts showing. They all know how long we have been waiting to have a baby. Whenever I feel sad, I tell myself, at least now I will be able to use my womb to feed my own baby.

Naseem's reproductive trajectory seems to be filled with ironies—from her attempts to have a second child to counter allegations of infertility, to the termination of the long-awaited pregnancy because of her husband's unemployment, and finally to her involvement in surrogacy. Naseem is 30 years old and is hopeful that she will be able to conceive a child of her own after the surrogacy birth.

Nisha, a 36-year-old surrogate for a couple from the United States, has accepted that she can no longer have more children of her own. She works as a nurse at the clinic. She decided to become a surrogate to pay for her husband's kidney operation:

> For the past two years I have been convincing other women to become surrogates and see now I am doing it myself! My husband refused in the beginning but there is so much money in just one year that he got convinced. I have just one son of my own and I always wanted one daughter but I don't think we would anymore. I know how much this takes out of your body. I've seen so many women go through this. I don't think at my age my body can take another pregnancy after this one.

The embodied nature of surrogacy as labor, and the multitude of bodily interventions it often requires, limits the number of possible pregnancies per woman. And in the trade-off between having another child of their own and having a child for money, surrogates like Parvati, Naseem, and Nisha choose the latter. By using terms like "trade-off" and "choice," I do not want to minimize women's pain in making these hard decisions. At the same time I do not want to naturalize or universalize maternal attachment and pain. In her thought-provoking book *Death Without Weeping: The Violence of Everyday Life in Brazil* (1992), Nancy Scheper-Hughes writes about mothers in a shantytown of drought-stricken Brazil. Scheper-Hughes contends that women in the shantytowns learn to economize grief and to accept the death of half their children not only as inevitable but as a blessing, as the best way to save the other half. She suggests that in a Euro-American context, mother love is culturally determined by the hegemonic biomedical model of maternal bonding, and this hegemonic model makes the experience of alternative maternal emotions seem unnatural (1992, 412). In the next section I discuss the surrogates' ambivalent responses to biomedicalization and counterintuitive portrayal of surveillance and medicalization as "luxuries they deserve." I demonstrate that these responses have to be situated within a particular social, cultural, and historical context. In the same way, the responses of surrogates to the trade-off between having their own pregnancy or having a surrogate pregnancy are contextual. While many surrogates choose to forgo having their own children out of sheer financial need, their actual responses ranged from casual acceptance to bitter resignation to fate. While some, like Naseem and Nisha, talk casually about their decisions to forgo having their own children and/or to get abortions, others, like Parvati, lament their fate.

THIS BIRTH AND THAT: NEGOTIATING THE "SCISSOR" (CAESAREAN SECTION)

Apart from the medications, injections, and weekly checkups during the initial months of pregnancy, the surrogates are subjected to another form of medical intervention: caesarean sections. Studies on biomedicalization and medical intervention in India have highlighted the "willingness" of women to subject themselves to such invasive techniques in order to make themselves "bioavailable" to the state, medical regime, and global markets (Cohen 2005; Van Hollen 2003).[7] This willingness is, allegedly, an effort to "remake one's mindful body in accordance with development modernity" (Cohen 2005, 87). In Garv, where health care, especially maternal health care, is unpredictable and difficult to access for most poor working-class women, "the time of bioavailability" was yet to arrive in 2006 but is being ushered in, rather abruptly, by the surrogacy industry (Pinto 2008, 15). Although most women had their previous deliveries at home with minimum medical intervention, as surrogates they inevitably undergo a caesarean section. Only two surrogates in this study had natural vaginal deliveries (see table 2). This development is partly an effort to accommodate the scheduling needs of the intended parents (especially international clients) and the scheduling needs of the clinic. The nurses hinted at another possible reason—the doctor's belief that the surrogate is likely to be less attached to the baby if the delivery is surgical. Desai is candid in his explanation: the higher chance of caesarean sections in surrogate births is because the babies are "precious."

> There is a higher chance of caesarean since *it's a precious baby*. Firstly, just the chances that a woman will get pregnant at all with someone else's child is so low, just 40 percent. On top of that, there are much higher chances of miscarriages in artificial birth. So once a surrogate does reach her last trimester successfully, we don't take any chances at the delivery stage and at the first warning signal we go for a caesarian. The surrogates don't mind, they are *willing* to do this for the sake of the baby [emphasis added].

While Desai asserts that the surrogates are willing, the "Scissor" (caesarean section) was a subject of much debate, negotiation, and sometimes resentment. Most surrogates used the English word "scissor" for caesarean sections. While some seemingly used it as an abbreviation of the unfamiliar English word "caesarean," others explained to me that they connected the surgery to cutting and hence "scissors." The use of the word "scissor" was very often accompanied by a two-finger gesture to indicate "cutting." Ramya, recovering from a caesarean (she delivered twins to the intended parents from the United States), talks candidly about the use and abuse of women's bodies throughout the surrogacy process, culminating in the "scissor":

> I came to the clinic the first time around two years ago. Since then I have been just in and out of this clinic. I don't ever want anyone else to go through this. It's not child's play. It's very painful—the medicines, the injections and now this scissor. It's not like there can't be normal [vaginal]

deliveries in this process but they [doctor and intended parents] don't want to take any risk. *The child is most important, not our bodies* [emphasis added]. But I cannot complain. Nature gave me a healthy body. I decided to let others cut it apart.

Ramya is well aware of the doctor's priority, the "precious baby," and contends that the high probability of a caesarean delivery is a clear indication of the unequal power relations in surrogacy—where the child born out of surrogacy is more valued than the health and welfare of the surrogate's body. But she simultaneously claims that since it was her "choice," she cannot complain. Ramya is one of the few to assert that surrogacy was her "choice."

Sharda had just delivered a baby to a couple from Mumbai, India, when I ran into her at the clinic. She looked very weak and underweight. A week later I see her walking a little with her husband's help, but she tells me she feels weak. She has no appetite or strength, but because the baby is underweight she has to feed him all the time. She is still on the catheter and tells me she had been bleeding excessively since the caesarean. Sharda starts talking about the delivery while breast-feeding the baby.

They [the nurses and the intended mother] keep scolding me because I am not eating enough. Sarita *didi* [the intended mother] is just worried about her son. She worries that I am producing such little milk that he has to pull harder. "How can a poor small thing pull so hard?" That's what she keeps saying. But what do I do, I feel too sick to eat. They made me have a *scissor*. I told them my first two children were normal, why do I need an operation now? I have lost so much blood. Ask my husband, he will tell you. I have become half my size. Just one [surrogacy] has done this to me. I know we will need more money again, but I am not sure I will be able to survive another one.

Like Ramya, Sharda is aware that the medical staff and the intended mother are anxious about postnatal nurture and nutrition not for her own sake but for the welfare of the "precious" baby. Her loss of appetite is a problem because she cannot produce enough breast milk for the baby. Although Ramya emphasizes her choice (in letting others cut apart her otherwise healthy body) more than Sharda does, both surrogates believe that the C-section is imposed and inevitable. Other surrogates, however, talk about their success in negotiating the level of biomedicalization of the birth process and their control over the ultimate nature of the delivery.

Rita has already delivered a baby to an Indian couple settled in the United States and is undergoing treatment to carry their second baby. She recalls the day of the delivery:

> I started having pains almost 15 days ahead of time but they gave me injections to let the pain subside. The doctors put me on some drugs because they wanted the delivery to happen only once the couple came down from America.
>
> I still remember the day of the delivery. They [the intended parents] started the day with a big *puja* [Hindu ritual]. They even took out a *muhurat* [auspicious time] for the delivery. I was so annoyed. Is there a good time for birth and death? I've been keeping this inside me for nine months and now you will tell me the time to get it out!

Rita is one of the two surrogates to have a vaginal delivery. This, she believes, is a result of successful negotiations with the intended parents and the doctors. "Once the *puja* was over, I told them that I want a normal delivery. They kept insisting that I should try for a scissor. But I did not give in. They made me wait for their convenience and I made them agree to a normal delivery for my convenience. I may want to do this [surrogacy] again later. If I had agreed to an operation, my chances of becoming a surrogate again would have decreased!"

Although most surrogates complain about the inevitable caesarean operation, especially since it reduces the possibility that they could become surrogates again, some assert that they actively chose a C-section over a natural delivery. Divya was carrying a baby for a couple from the United States when I met her for the first time, in 2006. She is an exception on many levels. A bank teller in the city, she is also the only college-educated surrogate at the clinic. In my second visit to the field, Divya recalls the day of the delivery. "Anne [the intended mother] came in on the eighth month and for two months she stayed with me. My blood pressure had been very high throughout my pregnancy, so I told Doctor Madam that I want a caesarean. I didn't want to take any risk with my health. My due date was a week later but I decided since my pressure was so high we should get him out sooner."

Divya is the only surrogate to demand a C-section. This could be partly because she is better educated than most other surrogates in this study and was more familiar with the medical system (she had already experienced a C-section). Although with varying degrees of success, some surrogates are able to negotiate with the doctor and have some control over the delivery process. While Divya asserts that she insisted on a C-section for the sake of her own health, all the other surrogates hoped for and/or demanded a vaginal birth. A vaginal birth not only meant fewer medical interventions but also increased the possibility that they could become surrogates again. These negotiations can be seen as labor-management strategies, used by the women in seeking to protect their own interests, although their definitions of "interests" often vary. Simultaneously, these victories give the women the feeling of being in control: of their bodies and their lives.

THIS BIRTH AND THAT: NEGOTIATING THE NATURE OF PRENATAL AND POSTNATAL CARE

The near inevitability of the C-section highlights the explicit power difference between client and surrogate, a clear manifestation of what feminist anthropologist Shellee Colen calls "stratified reproduction": power relations by which some categories of people are empowered to nurture and reproduce while others are disempowered (Colen 1995). While Colen used the term to compare the reproductive status of West Indian nannies to their (mostly) female employers, other scholars have adopted this term as a theoretical framework for examining a whole range of issues at the intersection of reproduction and stratification, including the use of assisted reproductive technologies (Ginsburg and Rapp 1991; Inhorn 2010; McCormack 2005; Twine 2011). Rayna Rapp expanded on the notion of stratified reproduction and defined it as the "hierarchical organization of reproductive health, fecundity, birth experiences, children, and child rearing that supports and rewards the maternity of some women while despising or outlawing the mother work of others" (Rapp 2001). Others have noticed this stratification specifically in the context of assisted reproductive technologies (Inhorn 2011; Twine 2011).[8] In her study of global surrogacy, sociologist France Winddance Twine (2011) reviews recent work (including my previous work on the topic) on commercial surrogacy in Egypt, Israel, India, and the United States, to argue that such stratification becomes exceptionally stark when the same women who are gestational surrogates for others are unable to afford basic health care when their contracts expire. Commercial surrogacy becomes "stratified contract labor" where the "economic benefits are structured along racial, ethnic and class lines" (15).⁹ Anthropologist Rayna Rapp calls this a reproductive hierarchy, where "some women struggle for basic reproductive technologies, like a clinic where sterile conditions might be available to perform C-sections, while others turn to cutting-edge genetic techniques" (quoted in Roberts 2009, 784). As the narratives and life experiences of surrogates at Armaan indicate, this stratification is indeed striking with regard to surrogacy in India—the same women who never had access to sterile clinics and C-sections are able to access it only as bodies that are facilitating other women's access to cutting-edge reproductive technologies.

The surrogates recognized and highlighted this stratification while comparing the experience of giving birth to their own children to the surrogacy birth process. But another parallel narrative is worth emphasizing. While most of the women candidly outlined the bodily interventions involved in the process of surrogacy (injections, medicines, tests, and surgeries), they simultaneously emphasized some practical advantages of biomedicalization and the "luxuries" it offers, albeit temporarily. Parvati compares her experience as a surrogate mother to her previous pregnancy:

> There is pain even with your own child. But with my own child, I did not understand what was going on with my body. I was too young; got married at the age of 16 and got pregnant with my son in just six months of getting married. This time is totally different. I am much more pampered, much more, say, in the know.
>
> The Doctor does not allow us to do any housework so I have hired a maid. I pay her with the money they [the intended parents] send every month. And since they want me to be strong and healthy, I eat lots of ice creams, coconut water, milk etc., every day. I pay for this out of the monthly cash. After all once the child is out, it's my body that will suffer and be weak if I don't eat healthy right now. I am supposed to take a lot of strength medicines [vitamins]. The doctor recommends one a day but I take two!

Parvati believes she is more in control of her surrogacy birth than she was for the birth of her own child. This is partly because in this pregnancy she is able to use the time to take care of herself, rest, and recover. She also manages to have some control over the medical interventions on her body. For instance, by taking more than the instructed dosage of vitamin pills, she seems to assert that she has better knowledge of her bodily needs than even the doctor does. Later in the conversation Parvati talks about the delivery: "Whether I join work or not will depend on the delivery. I told the Doctor I don't mind if it is a scissor. If it's normal I will rest for only six months. But I can rest for a whole year if it's a scissor. My husband thinks it's a little excessive; he thinks I am spending too much on myself. But I tell him, I know all this costs money but I deserve it."

Although Parvati does not negotiate the actual method of delivery (C-section or vaginal), she uses the hyper-medicalization of the surrogacy birth process partly to her advantage. She plans to use the time after surgery to take care of her body, and despite her husband's reluctance, she spends money on herself because she "deserves" it.

Razia is a 25-year-old mother of two and has been hired by a couple from California. She wants to build a house with the money she earns from the surrogacy. I meet Razia immediately after her C-section.

> I delivered yesterday—it was a scissor. My first two children were normal delivery at home. I have never come to a hospital before. Not even when I fell sick with typhoid! I was very scared when they told me I need a scissor. I am very scared of blood and injections. After the scissor, I decided I should make most of everything—God does everything for the best. I told her [the intended mother] that I want to rest for six months because of the operation. I also told her that I don't want to go home but rest at the clinic. And since we don't have extra money, I want them to pay for the extra months. They are very nice people, they agreed. With my own children I had to get back to backbreaking work almost the day they were out. *This time I can make it different* [emphasis added].

Although Razia is subjected to a C-section, she is able to negotiate extended postnatal care at the clinic. While after the birth of her own children she got no opportunity to recuperate, she believes that this time she can make her experience very different.

Regina is a 45-year-old surrogate in the ninth month of her pregnancy. Partly because of her age and possible complications in pregnancy, Regina has been instructed by the doctor to remain in the clinic till the time of her delivery. Regina talks about her life at the clinic:

> I know it will be a scissor, after all the medicines and injections that they have been feeding me, do you think the baby will come out that easily! I've been staying at the clinic for the past six months now. Doctor Madam

wanted me to stay here. And these nurses, they never leave me alone. Eat this, eat that, take this pill, don't walk so much. They even tell me whether I should bathe or not! I don't think even my mother worried so much when I was pregnant. With us it usually works like this: "Give birth, take a deep breath, get back to work."

Regina seems to have accepted the inevitability of the C-section as the final manifestation of the hyper-medicalization of surrogacy. At the same time, her response to the high level of everyday surveillance by the nurses and doctors is marked by ambivalence.

Of course, I don't like not being able to go home to my children. But I also don't mind staying here. Right now my son takes care of all the housework. But once I go back I will go back to being a mother, a house cleaner, a farmer, everything again! And it's not like I just work at home. I also clean other people's houses. All this [pampering] is my way of getting something back. Do you know, I sometimes ask my husband to give me a foot massage. I am sure he doesn't like that!

Although Regina resents not being able to visit her children, she relishes the opportunity to rest and get some reprieve from household and outside work. Parvati, Razia, and Regina are able to use the intense medicalization of the surrogacy birth process at least partly to their own advantage. Curiously, they also believe that they are much more in control of the surrogacy birth than they were for the birth of their own children.

At first glance it seems ironic that the women often frame the hyper-medicalization and surveillance of the birth process (typically assumed to be exploitative and restrictive) as "luxuries they deserve." This counterintuitive portrayal of medicalization and surveillance can be understood only within the historical context, in which most women in rural areas are exposed to a relatively low degree of biomedicalization of reproduction. Childbirth is treated as a routine occurrence, demanding little medical attention or care. The sudden professional care that they get as surrogates becomes "luxuries" that allow the women to take much better care of their health and their body. Unlike their earlier pregnancies and deliveries, the surrogate pregnancies not only involve better nutrition and medical care but also mean a reprieve from backbreaking work, an opportunity to spend some money on themselves, and a chance to take some time after the delivery to recuperate.

Other scholars have indicated similar paradoxical responses by economically disadvantaged women in other parts of South Asia and Africa. For instance, Ellen Gruenbaum (1998) argues that for the rural Sudanese women in her study the experiences of disempowerment are very different from those of women in the global north. She argues that people in the global north have experienced hyper-medicalization of many healthcare processes, which leads to a sense of disempowerment and a desire for alternatives. The economically disadvantaged and rural people in her study, however, often have a very different response to medicalization. It is often the *lack* of access to medical services that seems to constitute disempowerment for them. When viewed out of context, these responses may be interpreted simply as women colluding in their own oppression. Yet from another perspective, their responses may be a way to resist other forms of subordination.[10]

Inarguably, these small victories and the practical benefits that the women are able to incorporate into their everyday lives are essential pieces of the surrogacy story. But the bigger picture cannot be overlooked. It is important to highlight the fact that the women are able to negotiate better natal care only because the fetuses they are carrying enjoy higher social status. As lower-class women giving birth to lower-class babies, their own pregnancies are treated as everyday occurrences that do not deserve any prenatal or postnatal care and attention. As surrogates, however, they become wombs for "precious," middle-class, and international babies. Their bodies become only temporarily worthy of care because they are engaged in embodied labor whose purpose is to produce babies for rich(er) couples. In other words, the value of the child spills over unavoidably onto the bodies of the surrogates. The surrogates can then seize the opportunity to reinterpret the valuations to produce deserving selves.

BODY, LABOR, AND RESISTANCES

I started this chapter by lamenting that bodies seldom take center stage in the sociology of work, partly because of the historically gendered nature of work that involves use of the body. Most embodied forms of work are, thus, dismissed as "reproductive," outside the labor market and not visible as work at all. By analyzing surrogacy as an extreme example of the manifestation of worker embodiment, I challenge the gendered dichotomy between reproduction and production. The embodied labor tool not only challenges gendered dichotomies, but also allows us to examine the layers of domination and the multiple arenas of negotiations and resistances by the surrogates. On an everyday basis, the surrogates seem to be taking control of their bodies and lives by negotiating with their families (husbands and in-laws) and the clinic and by using their bodies for labor. At the micro-political level, these negotiations with the family are victories for women's self-esteem, providing them the ability to maneuver in their families and to make money by using the only resource they really have—their bodies.

As far as medicalization and resistance to the clinic are concerned, while some surrogates candidly acknowledge the magnitude of medical interventions, most do not resist them outright. Instead, they use their participation in this new form of embodied labor as a way to gain control over their bodies and reproduction, not just during the surrogacy process (for instance by negotiating the level of medicalization and postnatal care) but also beyond (by demanding vaginal delivery, by postponing sterilization, and by undergoing abortions of their own babies). The negotiations and resistances of these women need to be seen in light of the history of development of biomedicine in India. Most of these women have very little access to medical facilities and birth-related technology—typically they have home births with the help of midwives. In this context, for most surrogates, having access to prenatal, natal, and postnatal medical care and supervision becomes a "luxury" that they deserve for their "productive" motherhood. At the same time, most women in this study seem to have conflicting attitudes toward another imposed medical intervention—the caesarean section. While some resent the caesarean, partly because it reduces their chances of becoming a repeat surrogate, others use the prenatal, natal, and post-surgery-recovery period as a chance to rest, recover, and get some reprieve from everyday responsibilities.

The surrogates at Armaan are exerting control over their own bodies and lives by using their bodies for labor. The embodied labor performed by the surrogates subverts anti-natalist state propaganda and hegemonic narratives that frame the reproductive bodies of poor women as wasteful. At the risk of undermining the power of these subversive narratives, however, I urge readers to notice the unintended consequences of these resistances at the discursive and individual levels. In essence, individual resistances have unintended consequences whereby challenges to one form of domination almost inevitably lead to reification of another. Thus while the embodied labor that the surrogates undertake is an indication of creative resistance and of the ability of a group of women to convert their "wasteful" motherhood (as historically portrayed by the state) to productive motherhood (in terms of their ability to use their bodies to earn income), it is inherently paradoxical in nature. As these women align their own reproduction, through decisions about fertility, sterilization, and abortion, in order to (re)produce children of higher classes and privileged nations, they are fulfilling the global imperative of reducing the fertility of lower-class women in the global south.

Surrogacy in India is undoubtedly one of the clearest manifestations of stratified reproduction, where the fertility, bodies, and reproductive decisions of lower-class women become more valuable only insofar as these women serve as human incubators for their richer sisters. But classifying commercial surrogacy as stratified reproduction is too benign—as if the stratification happens by mere accident. Stratified reproduction in India, with surrogacy being one of its manifestations, is a result of conscious state priorities and an inevitable consequence of the present global division of both productive and reproductive labor. The Indian state remains determined to reduce the fertility of its lower-class citizens while at the same time it invests enthusiastically in technologically assisted reproduction of babies for its richer national and international clients through progressive medical tourism laws. In her study of the race-based reproductive hierarchy in the United States, legal scholar Dorothy Roberts eloquently comments: "The right to bear children goes to the heart of what it means to be human. The value we place on individuals determines whether we see them as entitled to perpetuate themselves in their children. Denying someone the right to bear children deprives her of a basic part of her humanity. When this denial is based on race, it also functions to preserve a racial hierarchy that essentially disregards Black humanity" (1997, 305). With the spread of new technologies to the global south, this racial hierarchy has been effectively globalized to disregard the humanity of women of color in the global south. Surrogacy in India is an explicit instance of this global reproductive hierarchy, or what I have termed "neo-eugenics." The neoliberal concept of unrestricted "consumer choice" teamed with the neoliberal understanding of the poor as "drains on the world's economy and society" becomes a convenient justification for this new form of eugenics. Feminist activist Betsy Hartmann sums it up concisely when she says: "[The surrogates in India] are literally producing citizens of other countries, while they remain second or third class citizens in their own, subject to a state-imposed two child norm when it comes to their own offspring" (2010, 6).

The body of the surrogate, however, is only one part of the disciplinary project, and correspondingly only one avenue through which the surrogates can negotiate, resist, and subvert. Just as critical to the disciplinary project is the production of the perfect mother-worker mind, especially the construction of the surrogate as a needy but not greedy mother, a disciplined yet disposable worker, and a loving yet disposable mother. But disciplinary strategies seldom go unchallenged. I devote the next chapter to the negotiation strategies used by the surrogates to challenge the medical and media construction of surrogates as dirty and disposable workers.

7 ✌ DISPOSABLE WORKERS AND DIRTY LABOR

FIELD NOTES, 2007, Armaan Maternity Clinic, Garv, India: The long room is lined with nine iron cots arranged with barely enough space to walk between them. It is rest hour at the hostel, so I walk up quietly to the last cot, where a 28-year-old widow, Yashoda, is resting after a surgery. She has been hired as a surrogate by a single man from Spain and was pregnant with triplets. One of the fetuses has just been surgically removed. She starts telling me her story—about her husband's death, and her neighbors abandoning "the widow who dared to become pregnant for some foreigner." When she breaks down in the middle and starts crying, the surrogate on the third bed gets up and completes Yashoda's story. By the end of the conversation eight of the nine are sitting around the bed, talking and listening. All agree that Yashoda need not feel guilty, that she has done nothing immoral. Surrogate Munni adds, "Go and tell your in-laws, 'At least I am not sleeping with anyone.'"

My early-morning conversations with the receptionist at the clinic involved drinking copious cups of tea, and, although I wasn't officially gathering data during those conversations, I unexpectedly found a rich source of information in my tea-drinking friend. Through those conversations, I learned that at any point in time, the number of clients waiting to be assigned a surrogate at the clinic was greater than the number of available surrogates. This reality made it even more critical that the disciplinary project convincingly establish the disposability of the women. This tactic worked in tandem with the constant yet contradictory use of the surrogate-prostitute analogy. As I discussed in chapter 4, the surrogate-prostitute comparison plays a critical role in the disciplinary project. The surrogate-prostitute analogy is selectively challenged or reinforced by the brokers, counselors, and medical professionals at different stages of the labor process. At the time of recruitment and counseling, the surrogates are assured that their role does not involve any "immoral acts" like having sex with clients. Nevertheless, in informal counseling and mentoring sessions, the "bad" surrogate, often the one who is business-minded and negotiates her wages, is compared to a prostitute. Consequently, the surrogate is under constant fear of crossing the thin line between morality and immorality. The surrogate stigma stems not only from the disciplinary project but also from broader perceptions of surrogacy in India. Like the whore stigma, the surrogate stigma reflects deeply felt anxieties about women trespassing the dangerous boundaries between private and public. Selling wombs for pay becomes an anomaly, much like selling bodies for pay.

Inarguably, commercial surrogacy, in which a woman agrees to waive her parental rights in exchange for payment, is a "cultural anomaly" (Teman 2006, 5). Although the anomalous process of surrogacy is an ethical quagmire in almost all countries, a critical reason for the huge amount of stigma surrounding surrogacy is that many Indians equate surrogacy with sex work. This conviction is partly the result of a lack of information—people are not aware of the technologies that can now separate pregnancy from sexual intercourse. The popular media add to this misconception, since almost all portrayals of commercial surrogacy in the media equate surrogacy with sex. One typical narrative is that of an infertile wife who agrees to bring a sex worker home to become impregnated by her husband through sexual intercourse. The alternative portrayal is of a sister/friend becoming a surrogate out of pure altruism and inevitably falling in love with the intended father.[1] Thus, all surrogates are portrayed as having some kind of "relation" (sexual or emotional) with the intended father of the child. Elsewhere, I have discussed surrogacy as "sexualized care work," a new type of reproductive labor that is similar to existing forms of care work but is stigmatized in the public imagination partly because of its parallels with sex work (Pande 2009b).

This stigma affects almost all the decisions made by the women at different stages of surrogacy. The clinic hires brokers and middle-women partly because women need convincing before they can be recruited into this stigmatized occupation. Once recruited, women often have no choice but to stay in the hostels and clinics, since many surrogates keep their surrogacy a secret from their community, their village, and very often their parents. Some decide to tell their neighbors the baby is their own and then later say that they had a miscarriage. A former surrogate, Sapna, explains why she decided not to tell even her parents: "My parents stay close by, but we didn't tell them. When it started showing we told them it is ours. When they asked us after the delivery how the baby was, we told them it had died. I am their daughter but still I think they'll misunderstand what I am doing. They'll think their daughter has been sleeping with an American."

Finally, this stigma and the subsequent separation from kin and community networks imply that the women have very little support from their kin and family during the nine months of pregnancy. Ramya has not revealed her pregnancy to anyone in her family, community, or village, and she is one of the few surrogates to recognize that the secrecy surrounding surrogacy and the subsequent isolation at the clinic and hostel make the surrogacy experience more painful:[2]

> Everyone thinks I am having his baby, our own baby. I had mentioned to people that my childless sister wants to adopt. When I go back home without a baby, I'll tell everyone that we gave away our child to my childless sister. I had to lie because people say so many bad things about surrogacy. They don't understand that we are not doing this for fun. You should make this point strongly in your paper, you should tell people, "Don't think badly of surrogate mothers, it just makes their pain even worse."

SURROGACY AS DIRTY WORK

The use of stigma as a tactic to exert discipline and control over women is not restricted to commercial surrogacy at the clinic. In many parts of the global south, young women are entering the workforce at a rapid rate, and they are thus exposed to and engage in activities that violate traditional boundaries in public life. As these women disrupt gender norms, they get constructed as deviants, responsible for the moral decadence of society. Management effectively uses this stigma to ensure compliance and maintain low pay. For surrogacy in Garv, however, the stigma has another benefit—it ensures that the women willingly stay at the hostel and subject themselves to an elevated level of surveillance.

The high level of stigma attached to surrogacy in India and the critical role it plays in the recruitment, discipline, and everyday negotiations by the surrogates themselves bring out fascinating parallels between commercial surrogacy and other forms of "dirty work." Work of various sorts has been classified as "dirty" because it seems to some to be "simply physically disgusting" (like janitorial work or butchering), it wounds one's dignity by requiring servile behavior (shoe shining, for example), or it in some way offends our moral conceptions (sex work, topless dancing, and surrogate mothering). In other instances, people may even applaud certain kinds of "tainted" or dirty work (like taking care of AIDS patients), but they "generally remain psychologically and behaviorally distanced from it" (Ashforth and Kreiner 1999, 416). Surrogacy work is similarly complex. Indeed, the literature on dirty work has argued that when individuals are engaged in a stigmatized occupation that threatens to "spoil their identity" it becomes necessary for them to do remedial work to control, manage, and neutralize the stigma associated with their deviant occupations (Goffman 1963; Sykes and Matza 1957). During the course of my fieldwork, I witnessed many kinds of remedial work done by the women to resist the stigma attached to surrogacy. These narratives largely denied the parallels between surrogacy and prostitution. But they simultaneously defied the medical construction of surrogates as disposable workers.

DRAWING MORAL BOUNDARIES: "WE ARE NOT BODY SELLERS OR BABY SELLERS"

Scholarship on identity work has contended that identity is defined relationally. For instance, British social historians and Birmingham School sociologists have considered how the working class defines its identity in opposition to those of other classes, or what sociologist Michele Lamont (2000) calls "boundary work"—constructing a sense of self-worth by interpreting differences between themselves and others. Holding oneself to high moral standards is also a way to acquire or affirm one's dignity at work. Often, this means defining the "others" as "low moral types" (Lamont 2000; Lamont and Fournier 1992). The literature on dirty work also indicates a similar pattern—members of dirty work occupations draw comparisons against salient occupational groups that they consider to be "somewhat similar in prestige but disadvantaged in some way. These groups are sufficiently similar to make the comparison believable but sufficiently "inferior" that it gratifies the need for self-esteem" (Ashforth and Kreiner 1999, 425). It is quite telling that the surrogates in my study often emphasized the moral difference between surrogacy and sex work and between surrogacy and putting a baby up for adoption. For the dirty workers of Garv, baby sellers (people who sold their genetic babies) and body sellers (women who had sex for money) were constructed as far more inferior and morally distant from the surrogates.

Meena's husband persuaded her to become a surrogate. He needed the money to pay the mortgage for his roadside barber stall. Meena accepts that she agreed to be a surrogate out of desperation, but emphasizes that her act of desperation was morally less tainted than stealing, murdering, or sleeping with someone: "I don't think there is anything wrong with surrogacy. We need the money and they need the child. The important thing is that I am not doing anything wrong for the money—not stealing or killing anyone. *And I am not even sleeping with anyone*" [emphasis added].

Dipali, a divorcée with three children, vocalizes her reason for not keeping her surrogacy a secret from her neighbors and parents—her work is less tainted than sex work: "I told my parents that I am doing this. I told them if you can help me, fine. But don't be a hindrance in what I am doing. If I was doing something wrong you could stop me, hit me, anything, but this is not wrong. At least I am not like some other women who have [sexual] relations for money, just because they are so desperate. This is what I told them."

Another kind of boundary work done by surrogates involves emphasizing the difference between giving a child away in surrogacy and giving a child away for adoption. Meena reasons that giving the child away right after birth will not be too difficult: "You have to weigh the pain with the need of the hour. We will at most cry for a week or two. But it would have been different if we had to give away our own child. No, we would never give away any of our real children. Only we know how we have raised them, taken care of them. *I don't understand how some people can do that*" [emphasis added].

Divya is carrying a baby for a couple from the United States. She also emphasizes the difference between surrogacy and giving away one's own child: "I think they [the intended parents] chose us because of Shalin [Divya's infant son]. He was very healthy then. They liked him so much that they wanted to just take him home with them! But we were sure about one thing, no one and nothing can make us give away our own child. *We are not like that. We won't sell our baby*" [emphasis in original].

Although putting up a child for adoption for money is hardly a norm in this region of India, surrogates constantly used this part-imaginary category of mothers as a way to establish their moral superiority. Yashoda, a widow and mother of three children, accepts that she constantly feels guilty for selling her womb, but she echoes Divya's assertion that "we are not like that. We won't sell our baby": "I know everyone feels pity and even revulsion for this desperate widow who is selling her womb. Yes, I will let you feel pity, let you call me desperate. But I will not allow you to call me a baby-seller. I have heard of women in situations like I am in, who end up doing the unthinkable. But however desperate I get, that is something I cannot even imagine doing . . . I will never sell my own children. What kind of a mother does that?"

Apart from morally distancing themselves from other groups of needy people, the surrogates sometimes used traditional morality to affirm their husband's dignity. In her study of working-class men in the United States, Lamont (2000) indicates how these men use religion to keep pollution at arm's length, including drugs, alcohol, promiscuity, and gambling, to draw boundaries against immoral men. In my study, the surrogates used similar techniques to vigorously defend their husbands' moral worth by comparing them to other men and other husbands—perhaps attempting to balance the moral stigma presumably attached to husbands who are not "man enough" to feed the family and who allow their wives to be pregnant for some other man.

Vidya is a 30-year-old surrogate and the mother of three children. She was persuaded by her sister-in-law to donate eggs at the clinic and then persuaded by the nurses to become a surrogate. "When I came here [the clinic] the first time they didn't really ask too many questions. They didn't have to check much either because he [her husband] is such a good person—doesn't drink, smoke anything. I am so lucky. Look everywhere, maybe not where you come from, but here husbands are very [laughs] like bulls. But my husband has never raised his hand at me."

Anjali, a thin woman in her early twenties, has no idea about the money involved in the contract or the exact medical procedures. Her husband seems to be the one in control of the finances. Like Vidya, she was also persuaded by her sister-in-law to donate eggs at the clinic and then persuaded by the nurses to become a surrogate. Anjali accepts that she is desperate for the money. During the time of the interview she was breast-feeding her own baby. She had to persuade Dr. Khanderia to allow her to be a surrogate even though she was still breast-feeding because there was no money in the house to buy milk for the baby—her husband has no permanent job and she is a housewife. "My husband is unemployed but he is a very good person. He takes care of the children. He stays at home mostly so he knows what to feed them. Most husbands would not agree to let their wives do this [be a surrogate], but he agreed. I am very lucky. We had no issues [with getting the surrogacy contract] because his history is so clean. He doesn't smoke or drink. We are Christians. He converted [from Hinduism] and used to work in a Mission earlier."

The surrogates in my study resist the stigma of surrogacy by constructing a sense of self-worth and by interpreting differences between themselves and other just as needy but "less moral types" like body-sellers and baby-sellers. Simultaneously, through these discursive strategies, they uphold the morality of their husbands. The surrogates emphasize the religiosity of their husbands and the absence of any vices, presumably to resist the stigma attached to men who cannot provide for their wives and for that reason allow them to become pregnant for someone else.

DOWNPLAYING THE ASPECT OF CHOICE: "THIS IS NOT WORK, THIS IS *MAJBOORI* (A COMPULSION)"

Ironically, while supporters of surrogacy emphasize the element of choice in surrogacy (i.e., that a woman has the right to choose what to do with her body), most of the surrogates' narratives indirectly downplay choice as part of their decision, as if to say, "It was not in my hands, so I cannot be held responsible, and should not be stigmatized." One of the ways the surrogates justify their decision is to emphasize that surrogacy is not work but a compulsion. Salma is a surrogate for clients from the United States. Unlike Dipali and Meena, Salma accepts that she believes surrogacy is unethical but emphasizes that it is an act of survival and necessity— because prestige alone will not "fill an empty stomach":

Who would choose to do this? I have had a lifetime's worth of injections pumped into me. Some big ones in my hips hurt so much. In the beginning I had about 20–25 pills almost every day. I feel bloated all the time. But I know I have to do it for my children's future. *This is not work, this is* majboori *[a compulsion]* [emphasis in original]. Where we are now, it can't possibly get any worse. [She uses a local proverb:] We don't have a hut to live in or crops in our farm to fill our stomach with.

This surrogacy is not ethical—it's just something we have to do to survive. When we heard of this surrogacy business, we didn't have any clothes to wear after the rains—just one pair that used to get wet—and our house had fallen down. What were we to do? Let me tell you something, there are many families like ours who want to do it, but either the husband doesn't approve or the wife doesn't agree to do it. These people are jealous. These are the kind of people who call it immoral. And if everyone in the family agrees, society disapproves. But I say if your family is starving what will you do with respect? Prestige won't fill an empty stomach.

Apart from emphasizing their *majboori* in making the decision to become surrogates, the surrogates also appeal to higher loyalties, by emphasizing that they would be using the money not for self but for family, especially children. Anjali defends her decision to become a surrogate: "I am doing this basically for my daughters—both will be old enough to be sent to school next year. I want them to be educated, maybe become teachers or air hostesses? I don't want them to grow up and be like me—illiterate and desperate. I don't think there is anything wrong with surrogacy. But of course people talk. They don't understand that we are doing this because we have a compulsion. People who get enough to eat interpret everything in the wrong way."

Vidya, another surrogate, echoes Anjali's sentiment: "I am doing this basically for my children's education and my daughter's marriage. We have lived our life, we have survived it. But they should grow up happier. I want them to grow up and be proud of their parents. I want them to be educated so that in case anything happens to us they can take care of themselves. I am doing everything for them. I am not greedy for the money."

It is worth noting that the families of the surrogates also downplay the degree of choice that the surrogate has, in addition to differentiating surrogacy from other kind of occupations. Surrogacy, the men in the family argue, is more like a "calling," God's blessings that would enable a woman to fulfill her familial obligations. Parag compares his wife Meena's surrogacy to *tapasya*—the Hindu principle and practice of physical and spiritual austerity and discipline to achieve a particular aim: "I don't think this is work. When you became a teacher, you just went ahead, took your exams and became a teacher. This is not like that. It is like God helped her do this for our family. It is like praying to God—like *tapasya*. This is her prayer to God and ultimately she will get his blessings and her dreams will be fulfilled. Like saints pray under austere conditions, she is living here in the clinic, getting all those injections, going through all this pain. But she will get the fruit of her labor."

Alternatively, surrogacy is portrayed as a "team effort" made by the entire family to improve their financial situation, a view that ignores the critical gendered nature of this work, that it is only the woman doing all the body and emotion work. The husbands and in-laws often speak of surrogacy not as individual (woman's) choice or work but as a team effort. Sapna has decided not to become a surrogate again. She has delivered twins for a couple from America, and the money earned is being spent on building a house for the family. But her father-in-law, Manoj, feels cheated and complains, "Even though everyone delivers one and *we* delivered two babies—still we got the same rate. They should have paid *us* more. That's why *we* decided we would not do it again. We lost our respect in society and didn't even get paid enough for it" [emphasis added].

In their analysis of gestational surrogacy in India, DasGupta and Das DasGupta (2010) persuasively argue that in South Asian societies, the language of individualism, autonomy, and ownership has little resonance. Instead, there is an emphasis on the "relational" and collective. In such contexts, "one's body is not one's own but the responsibility of the collective" (140). Lesley Sharp (2000) and Rosalind Petchesky (1995) have provided similar cautions against universalizing the "Western and capitalist" preoccupations with body as property, and the right to autonomous ownership of this body. But what is worth mentioning is that while the male members of the family enthusiastically appropriate this language of collective ownership and team spirit, the surrogates themselves are more ambivalent. As discussed in chapter 6, for some surrogates, using their bodies for work *is* a way to emphasize their ownership over their bodies. Others frame their ownership of body more in the context of their past inability to make any decisions regarding their sexuality and reproduction. Still others reiterate their substantial and labored contribution toward the process to undermine the relative contribution of male members. This will be examined in more detail in chapter 8. At the same time, however, most surrogates continue to give relational—not individual—rationales for taking part in surrogacy. Surrogacy is undertaken as a sense of familial duty, out of economic desperation and not as an occupation of choice.

Surrogates use the language of morality and moral boundaries to affirm their dignity and sense of self-worth, in turn reducing the stigma attached to surrogacy. Additionally they, along with their families, downplay the element of choice—by highlighting their economic desperation, by appealing to higher motivations, or by emphasizing the role of a higher power (God) in making the decisions for them. Ironically, while these narratives resist the dominant discourse of surrogates as "dirty workers," they reinforce certain gender hierarchies. Feminist scholars have argued that motherhood reifies the identity of women as primarily relational and bound by duties to others (Jeffery 2001). This is reflected in the narratives used by the surrogates. The "lack of choice" and "higher loyalties" narratives reinforce the image of women as selfless dutiful mothers whose primary role is to serve the family, their husbands, and their in-laws. Similarly, the emphasis on the "high morality" of their husbands and their "generosity" in giving permission to their wives to be surrogates indicates that the women may be overcompensating for their (temporary) role as breadwinners.

DENYING DIRT AND DISPOSABILITY: "IF WE ARE ALL JUST DIRTY WOMBS, WHY ARE WE PAID DIFFERENT AMOUNTS?"

In her book *Disposable Women and Other Myths of Global Capitalism*, Melissa Wright (2006) provides a powerful analysis of the "myth of disposability" of women workers in global factories. She argues that it is the inherent "paradox" of this myth that "provides it with organizational structure"—the Third World woman is assumed to be easily substitutable and yet is simultaneously believed to possess the exact qualities (dexterity and patience) that make her invaluable. This "internal contradiction" is exactly what makes this myth a "socially useful lie" that can be used to "influence social behavior on the basis that power is naturalized, apolitical and beyond human intervention" (2006, 4). This myth effectively works as a disciplinary mechanism by defining the behavior expected from a "normal" disposable Third World woman. As discussed in chapter 4, a similar trope of disposability permeates the lives of womb workers at Garv in the form of disciplinary tactics that aim to manufacture the perfect mother-worker mind and body. These discourses, however, do not go unchallenged. Some surrogates emphasize their own "special" qualities that make couples choose them over all the other surrogates. Others stress the "special" quality of the hiring couple and the exceptional bond they share with the couple.

Puja, the repeat surrogate introduced earlier, challenges the notion of a surrogate's disposability:

If we are all just dirty wombs, why are we paid different amounts? I am getting much more than many of the surrogates here. An Indian couple came from America during the delivery of my first baby. They said that they don't care how long they have to wait—I can rest for one, two years, as much as I want, but they only want me to carry their baby. Mrs. Shah—the woman—she is also a Brahman [upper caste]. Maybe that's why she liked me, because I am clean. But almost everyone who comes here for a surrogate wants me. Doctor Madam says to me, "Why can't you get me ten, fifteen more Pujas!"

Puja mentions the relatively higher pay offered to her to argue that she is special. She believes that couples want her to bear their children partly because she is of a higher caste and "clean." Other surrogates made similar claims to establish their indispensability. Divya, a former surrogate, proudly relates her first encounter with potential clients, when she rejected the clients that wanted to hire her: "There was another couple from Delhi that we were introduced to first. But we somehow didn't like them. They didn't seem to have any love for Shalin [Divya's infant son]. You need to have love for children before you decide to come in and look for a surrogate. We took a risk but we said no to them. Dr. Khanderia was surprised because it's usually the couples who reject surrogates."

Divya is an exception on many levels, and her story is unusual. There are no other instances that I am aware of where the surrogate refused a client. Divya is the only surrogate with a college education and also the only one who is not from that region. All other surrogates in the clinic are from nearby villages, but Divya has traveled from a distant metropolitan area. This, she feels, increases her negotiating power and also makes her more special than "one of the other girls."

"Anne [the intended mother] wants two more children and in December she will get another surrogate," Divya says. "Of course she wanted me but I have already had two caesarean babies. I know how sad she is feeling that this time she will have to just get one of these other girls to be her surrogate."

The "I am special" narrative seems exceptionally powerful when invoked by lower-class women in India—a country in which sex-selective abortions, skewed sex ratios at birth, high female infanticide and mortality, and the use of ultrasound and amniocentesis during pregnancy present compelling evidence of the extensive prevalence of son preference. The feeling of "being special," albeit transient, affects the surrogates' perception of self-worth. Puja, who believes that she is the "most-wanted" surrogate, adds, "My husband feels proud of me. Well, he should. I have earned so much money and done something that even he couldn't have. Although he doesn't want me to do it again I think I would. I want to keep some money in a fixed account for my old age."

Puja is one of the few women to challenge narratives, related by male members of the surrogates' families, that surrogacy is a team effort. She constantly emphasizes that she has earned the money and she will decide what to do with it. Later in the conversation she talks about her dream to go abroad: "You know I had always dreamt of being an air hostess. But when I saw the situation at home—with my father earning only Rs. 1,500—I knew I couldn't study anymore. I just wanted to see America once, so badly. Once I got married I thought it would never happen. But now that I am planning to do this [surrogacy] for the second time, I feel why not? If I can do this here, maybe I can get some job there as well, no?"

Thus, for some surrogates, the narrative of "being special" did more than just counter the stigma of being dirty or disposable workers; it encouraged them to think of their own needs and it increased their self-esteem.

Apart from stressing their own "special" qualities, a complementary narrative used by the surrogates was that their clients were unique. Although most clients hiring a surrogate tried to build some kind of a relationship with her, the rules of commercial surrogacy meant that the termination of that relationship was rather abrupt. Dr. Khanderia ensured that the baby was taken away right after delivery so that the surrogate had no opportunity to change her mind. Several of the surrogates, however, reiterated how the couple hiring them was different and would not adhere to the clinic rules. Divya talks lovingly about Anne, the intended mother of the baby: "Most couples take away the baby right after delivery—these are the rules of this place. But Anne is not like that. She will come here with the baby and stay with me. She told me that I could rest in this apartment [that the hiring couple pay for] after delivery for a month if I want to."

Divya shows me the toys Anne has sent from the United States for Divya's infant son, Shalin. "We are very lucky. No one has got a couple as nice as ours. It's not just because she is a white lady that I say that. She has become such a close friend that if she calls us we'll even go visit her in Los Angeles and now we won't have to worry about staying in a hotel. I am sure they will take care of Shalin's health education, everything." Divya believes that by building a long-lasting friendship with the couple she has secured not just a plane ticket to California but also her son's future.

Regina is pregnant for an Indian couple settled in Dubai. Like Divya, she talks lovingly about the intended parents:

They are really nice people and call me *didi* [elder sister]. I call her [the intended mother] younger sister. She is younger than me. She is not from here but she feels like my own sister. She always worries about me, how I am doing, whether I am eating enough. She can't speak Hindi so she calls up Divya *didi* to find out about my health. We have started loving each other like family. They keep saying that they will remain indebted to me forever. I know they will stay in touch with me even after the delivery.

The surrogates resist the commercial and contractual nature of their relationship by establishing a relationship with their clients. Although they recognize the immense class difference between the couple and them, they sometimes construct relationships in their narratives that transcend the transnational and class differences. Thus the surrogates are able to construct kinship and friendship connections, whether real or imaginary, with women from outside their class and sometimes outside their national boundaries. Improvising within preexisting structural and cultural constraints, surrogate mothers manage to construct a relationship of sorts with the client and reinforce their self-worth. In chapter 8 I discuss in more detail the repercussions of these real or fictive kin ties forged with the intended mother. But one of the direct consequences of such a connection is the detrimental effect on the surrogates' ability to negotiate payment. While the ties forged by the surrogates can be seen as a form of resistance to medical narratives and procedures that underscore the surrogates' disposability, such relationships between surrogates and intended parents make the remuneration structure even more informal, often to the detriment of the surrogates. In the absence of any binding law or contract, individual couples have considerable freedom in deciding not just the boundaries but also the form of remuneration. A couple from New Jersey, for example, decided to pay the entire amount in kind to their surrogate, Salma. Salma explains: "Will [the intended father] said, 'You make us happy and we'll make you happy.' His wife has become like an elder sister to me so I do just want to see them happy. They said they would build a house for us wherever we want to build it and however big we want it to be. I am having twins so perhaps they will build us two rooms instead of one. But I don't want to ask."

The surrogates are reluctant to talk about the contract and the payment that they believe they deserve, in part because of the "special" ties forged with the clients, particularly with the intended mother. Teman (2010, 209) reports similar repercussions of the surrogate–intended mother relationship—the "tyranny" of this relationship forces the surrogate to go beyond contractual obligations. But for the surrogates at Armaan, the reluctance to negotiate payments is also shaped by the disciplinary discourses used in the clinic and hostel, and the different ways that the mother and the worker components of the dyad are dealt with in these discourses. While there is a lot of explicit discussion about good and bad motherhood, the construction of workers goes almost unspoken, concealing the commercial aspect. In chapter 4 I discussed that the consequent dual construction of surrogates as "mother-workers" has a corollary that a surrogate must be a good mother before she can be a good worker. This not only creates surrogates that are ideal for national and international clients, but it also inhibits the women from identifying as wage-earning workers. Ironically, the narratives that resist the clinic's construction of surrogates as dirty and disposable workers and instead emphasize their moral worth ultimately undermine their identity as workers and as wage earners for their own families.

REMEDIAL WORK AND DISCURSIVE RESISTANCE: A TOOL OF SUBVERSION?

In this chapter, my primary motivation has been to analyze the resistive practices of commercial surrogate mothers in India in a context shaped by both the relations of medical and global commoditization of women's bodies and the cultural stigmatization of women who use their bodies and wombs to work. While the narratives of the surrogates ostensibly work toward just remedying the stigma attached to surrogacy, they simultaneously resist certain subject positions assigned to the women by dominant discourses, especially the "myth of disposability" advanced by the clinic.

It is no surprise that the various stakeholders, from family members to medical staff, attach a variety of meanings to surrogacy that position the surrogates as subjects within the process. The media and the community often equate surrogates to sex workers. The medical staff often appropriates the prostitute-surrogate analogy to discipline the surrogates. Simultaneously, the surrogates' husbands and in-laws view surrogacy as a familial obligation, and not as labor performed by the women. A third kind of meaning attached to the role of surrogates lies in the medical narratives, in which surrogacy is perceived as an impersonal contract and surrogates as disposable workers. In the counseling sessions, the surrogate's transience and dispensability as both a worker and a mother are highlighted. These discourses do not go unchallenged. The surrogates resist the idea of disposability by forging relations with the intended mother. Some surrogates emphasize the "special" quality they have that made the clients choose them over all the other workers. Others focus more on the "special" quality of their clients and the exceptional bond they share with each other. But how relevant are these covert and symbolic forms of resistance? While the surrogates' language of morality affirms their dignity and sense of self-worth and reduces the stigma attached to surrogacy, it ultimately reinforces certain gender hierarchies. Ironically, while the focus of this study has been on surrogacy as labor, most surrogates do not speak of surrogacy as work that they have chosen. It is almost as if the surrogates do not resist the image of women as selfless dutiful mothers whose primary role is to serve the family. Similarly, their vigorous defense of their husbands' moral worth indicates that the women are overcompensating for their (temporary) role as breadwinners.

Discursive resistance has the potential to both transform and reproduce power relations, and to both resist and reaffirm subject positions. The clear emphasis in the surrogates' narratives on their clients' "special" quality is an example of this tension. Although the narratives used by surrogates to minimize the feeling of disposability and the stigma attached to being disposable workers seem powerful when invoked by lower-class women in India, the dream of a wealthier/white family coming to rescue them from desperate poverty and a bleak future brings in new forms of subjection based on race and class domination. Simultaneously, these (often fictive) relationships formed with intended parents downplay the contractual and commercial aspect of surrogacy, further undermining the surrogates' ability to view themselves as breadwinners as well as to defend their interests as workers.

The peculiarity of surrogacy is that the surrogates' identity as workers is intimately connected with their identity as mothers. Just as the clinic employs this dual identity to its own benefit, the surrogates themselves constantly negotiate the duality on an everyday basis. In this chapter I focused on the discursive strategies of the surrogates as they grapple with the stigma of being *disposable and dirty workers*. Chapter 8 brings into the conversation the other part of the puzzle—the surrogates' negotiation of the medical construction of surrogates as *disposable mothers*.

8 ✍ DISPOSABLE MOTHERS AND KIN LABOR

Anne [the intended mother from the United States] wanted a girl but I told her even before the ultrasound, coming from me it will be a boy. My first two children were boys and this one will be too. And see I was right it is a boy! After all she just gave the eggs, but the blood, all the sweat, all the effort is mine [emphasis added]. Of course it's going after me.

—Divya, a gestational commercial surrogate in Garv, 2006

IN SURROGACY, nothing guarantees one's status as the parent: not eggs, sperm, womb, or breast milk. From the famous 1986 Baby M case in New Jersey, in which the surrogate mother refused to return the baby girl to the intended parents[1] to the more recent 2008 Baby Manji case in Gujarat, in which both Indian and Japanese authorities refused to recognize the Japanese biological father as the real father of the baby born out of surrogacy,[2] many custody cases have been fought over whether the genetic mother, the gestational mother, the egg donor, or the genetic father has rightful claim to the baby. In fact, several ART clinics like Armaan Maternity actively discourage traditional surrogacy because they assume that when the same woman provides the egg and the womb she is more likely to renege on the contract and make claims on the baby. Dr. Khanderia's perfect mother-workers, however, have remained true to the management and as of the publication of this book no surrogate at Armaan Maternity Clinic has demanded custody of the baby. But legal battles are just part of the story. How do the surrogates negotiate these fraught relationships on an everyday basis?

According to classic kinship studies, kin relations are grounded in "natural" (read: biological) ties that supposedly make them immutable, special, and distinct from relationships formed in other ways (such as adoption or shared residence). Anthropologist David Schneider (1984) was among the first scholars to challenge traditional assumptions about biological kin relations. He demonstrated that kinship theory based on Euro-American folk assumptions about the primacy of procreative ties did not necessarily apply across cultures. In the last few decades many scholars have destabilized the essentialist and naturalized assumptions of kinship studies by emphasizing the *context* of these relations (Carsten 2000; Levine 2003; Peletz 1995; Schneider 1984; Strathern 1992; Thompson 2005).[3] Surrogacy, especially gestational surrogacy, in which someone else's fertilized eggs are implanted in the surrogate, provides a perfect opportunity to destabilize any assumptions around kin ties and instead pay attention to the "paradox" and "ambivalence" in kin ties (Peletz 1995, 360). This reproductive option, for instance, creates three possible categories of mothers: the biological mother (the woman who contributes the ovum), the gestational or womb mother (the surrogate), and the social or adoptive mother (the woman who raises the child) (Ragoné 1994, 111).

Scholars have previously discussed the many ways by which surrogate mothers negotiate their ties with the fetus, as well as with the intended mother (Ragone 1994; Teman 2010). But for the surrogates living in isolation in surrogacy hostels, with little interaction with their family and minimal interaction with the intended mother, the kin ties forged take on a whole new meaning. While the disciplinary project, the surveillance, and the clinic rules disrupt their existing relationship with their own husbands and children, this same project encourages the surrogates to seek and create networks and creative ties outside of the mainstream. Women respond to the medical construction of surrogates as disposable mothers by forging kin ties with the baby, the intended mothers, and other surrogates. Building on Micaela di Leonardo's concept of "kin work" (the work required to maintain cross household kin ties), I use the term "kin labor" to capture the whole range of labor performed by the surrogates, including gestation, giving birth, maintaining ties with the intended mother after birth, and forming a supportive community with the other surrogates at the clinic and hostel.[4] In the narratives of surrogates the kin labor manifests as both "*khoon paseena*" (the metaphor sweat-blood often used for hard labor) of maintaining kin ties and, more specifically, *khoon aur paseena* (sweat and blood of giving birth). Just as powerfully, these ties based on the kin labor done by different actors involved in surrogacy often take precedence over traditional bases of kin ties.

"WHATEVER EVERYONE SAYS, I AM NOT A BAD MOTHER": MOTHERS IN HIDING

Before turning to the surrogates' construction of new kin relationships, it is important to recognize how the process of surrogacy alters the women's existing kin ties. For the women at Armaan, relationships with husbands and children were directly affected by their contractual obligations as surrogates. In some cases it meant being away from home for nine months or more. For other surrogates who were allowed to return home, the doctor mandated that their domestic duties and mothering responsibilities be significantly reduced. For instance, women were instructed not to bend down to mop, wash clothes, or even lift an infant child. While most husbands visited their wives regularly, children were rarely seen at the hostel, especially since many surrogate mothers kept their surrogacy a secret from their children.

Scholarship on migrant women has discussed at length the effects of long distance "transnational motherhood" on a woman's relationship with her children left back at home (Gamburd 2000; Hondagneu-Sotelo and Avila 1997; Parreñas 2005). For instance, in their work on Latina migrant mothers, Pierrette Hondagneu-Sotelo and Ernestine Avila beautifully illustrate the way globalization and the flow of caregivers from the global south to the north build alternative constructions of motherhood. These alternatives do not conform to either the middle-class white ideal of motherhood in the United States or the Latina ideal. Transnational mothers use different mechanisms to legitimize these alternatives: they expand their definition of motherhood to include breadwinning and emphasize the positive impacts of their incessant communication and long-distance guidance in their children's lives. Their coping mechanisms also include bonding with their employer's children as if they were their own and being critical of their employer's "neglectful" parenting. Much like the women in the migration literature, surrogate mothers negotiate their new identity as primary breadwinners of the family rather than primary caregivers to their own children in different ways.

Puja is a surrogate for the second time in two years. She used the money earned from her first surrogacy contract to buy a small piece of land. She hopes to buy another piece of land with her second surrogacy and give that land as dowry at her daughter's wedding. She reiterates constantly that she is not a "bad mother":

> Doctor Madam had told me I could go home since I am very healthy. But I thought, why go home? At home I will have to clean, cook everything.

Here, the couple will pay for my food. My husband is not very happy, but I told him I deserve this rest. I miss my children, yes. I am not a bad mother. Which mother can do so much, you tell me? I have already bought a piece of land and will buy another one with this one [surrogacy]. It's not for me, she [her daughter] will get that as dowry. I am not at home, yes, but that is for now. I am giving more than any other mother can. Whatever everyone says, I am not a bad mother.

Later in the conversation Puja reveals that she has not told her children that she is a commercial surrogate. Her eight-year-old son overheard someone talking about Puja's pregnancy and was very disturbed. Puja accepts that the secrecy surrounding her surrogacy is difficult for her children, but she believes that it is her husband's responsibility to manage the situation at home: "He [her son] must have heard it from somewhere and he, poor boy, went and told everyone at school that his mother is pregnant and will get money for that. And of course his friends teased him and he came home crying. But what can I do? I am already handling a lot of things here. I know this thing is very strange for them [both of her children] and they are bothered by this mystery, but he [her husband] has to deal with it. I can't do everything."

Puja believes that she is compensating for her absence from home by fulfilling the material needs of her children. She recognizes the ill effects that the "mystery" surrounding surrogacy has on her children, but she simultaneously asserts that her husband needs to take responsibility for ensuring their mental well-being since she is managing their monetary well-being .

Dipali is a divorcée with two children. Unlike Puja, Dipali decided to discuss everything frankly with her children. "I told them, your mother is doing this for you, like this. I am not ashamed of this. My brother takes care of everything now. But things have to change when things have to change, no? I am doing something I never thought I would. My children will miss me now, but they will understand why I did it later, when they grow up and then they will thank me."

Surrogates like Puja and Dipali feel some level of guilt in their new identity as absent mothers, but also a sense of pride in their accomplishment. Both Puja and Dipali advocate for a broader conceptualization of good mothering that includes material provision and not just active care work. In their attempt to negotiate the contradictory demands of surrogacy and the hostel regime, surrogates not only redefine their relationship with their own children but also construct new kin ties with the baby born from the surrogacy.

"IT MAY BE HER EGGS, BUT IT'S MY SWEAT AND BLOOD": REDEFINING THE BLOOD TIE

Recent works on kinship have acknowledged that the boundaries between the social and the biological are "more permeable" in people's local discourses and "indigenous practices of relatedness" than what was assumed by classic kinship studies (Carsten 2000, 10). While dominant discourses emphasize the immutable father-child blood tie, ties are more fluid in local idioms like "shared bodily substances" (Daniel 1984; Lambert 1996, 2000; Strathern 1988). The relative contributions of mother and father are also expressed in terms of these substances—semen, blood, and milk.[5] For instance, in the textual and oral traditions of people in India, there is a strong emphasis on the father's contribution to procreation (Böck and Rao 2000; Hershman 1981). At one level there is recognition that bodily substances, like blood and breast milk, are shared between mother and child. These shared substances are assumed to establish automatic ties between mother and fetus, but do not trump the contribution of semen. A strong patrilineal focus can be seen, for instance, in the notions of "seed" and "earth," where seed symbolizes the father's contribution and earth or field represents the role of the mother (Dube 1986; Khare 1992). The (male) seed remains the accepted essence for creation of an offspring while women are expected to behave like earth, receive the male seed and give back the fruit, preferably male children (Dube 2001; Fruzzetti and Östör 1984; Madan 1981; Meillassoux 1981). Simultaneously, since in local idioms as well as in the indigenous system of medicine, *Ayurveda*, semen is assumed to originate from blood, a child becomes not just a product of the father's seed, but is also assumed to "inherit the *father's blood* and is therefore placed in his group" (Kumar 2006, 289). Female bodily fluids merely nourish the fetus but do not impart identity to a child (Fruzzetti and Östör 1984). As Fruzzetti and Östör succinctly put it, "[B]lood is male, and while it is unchangeable, it is transmitted in the male line and cut off at some point in the female line" (1984, 103). The surrogates at Armaan, however maintain a very different interpretation of the blood tie. They not only claim that the fetus is nourished by its *gestational* mother's blood but also emphasize that this blood/substance tie imparts *identity* to the child. Women within the surrogacy process are more than mere receptacles of male seed.

Parvati, hired by a couple from Mumbai, is 36 and one of the oldest surrogates at the clinic. I meet Parvati immediately after she had undergone a fetal reduction procedure. She tells me that she was against the surgery: "Doctor Madam told us that the babies wouldn't get enough space to move around and grow, so we should get the surgery. But both Nandini *didi* [the genetic mother] and I wanted to keep all three. We had informally decided on that. I told Doctor Madam that I'll keep one and *didi* can keep two. *After all it's my blood even if it's their genes* [emphasis added]. And who knows whether at my age I'll be able to have more babies."

Parvati thus uses her interpretation of the blood tie—"it's my blood even if their genes"—to make claims on the baby. Divya makes a similar claim. But in addition to the substantial ties of blood, Divya also emphasizes the *labor* of gestation and giving birth—her "sweat" ties with the baby—as another basis for making claims on the baby. I bump into Divya right after her second ultrasound, and she tells me, "Anne, the woman from California who is hiring me [the genetic mother], wanted a girl but I told her even before the ultrasound, coming from me it will be a boy. My first two children were also boys. This one will be too. And see, I was right, it is a boy! After all *they just gave the eggs, but the blood, all the sweat, all the effort is mine. Of course it's going after me* [emphasis added]."

This sweat (labor) and blood (substance) tie between surrogate and fetus is often advocated by the surrogates as being stronger than a connection based solely on genes. Sharda is one of the few surrogates who also breast-fed the baby that she delivered. This, she feels, intensifies her ties with the baby.

> I am not sure how I feel about giving the baby away to her [the genetic mother]. I know it's not her fault that she could not raise her own baby [in her womb] or breast-feed him. She has kidney problems. But she does not seem to have any emotional ties or affection for him either. Did you see when the baby started crying, she kept talking to you without paying him any attention? She keeps forgetting to change his nappies. Would you ever do that if you were a real mother? When he cries I want to start crying as well. It's hard for me not to be attached. I have felt him growing and moving inside me. I have gone through stomach aches, back aches and over five months of loss of appetite! I have taken nearly 200 injections in my first month here. All this has not been easy.

According to Sharda, her substantial ties with the baby (blood and breast milk) as well as the labor and effort she has put in to gestate the baby makes her more attached to it than the genetic mother is. Much like the transnational migrant mothers criticized their employers' "neglectful mothering" as a way to legitimize their long-distance mothering, Sharda criticizes the genetic mother's lack of concern for the newborn baby. Sharda believes that since the genetic mother has not put in the labor of gestation and giving birth she is incapable of feeling the emotions of a "real" mother.

Diksha, like Sharda, was one of the few surrogates "permitted" to breast-feed the baby. Diksha's story is unusual. Her Japanese clients had trouble arranging the legal papers required to take the baby back home and requested that Diksha take care of the baby in the interim period. For two months Diksha looked after the baby under the doctor's supervision. Diksha talks of her "daughter" with a smile on her face:

> She is my first baby girl. I have two sons and I always craved for a girl. *I know she looks Japanese, but I think of her as my own daughter* [emphasis added]. Well, it was different for me. I had her with me for not just the nine months [of pregnancy] but even after that. The two months we had her with us, I pampered her, you don't know how much! I splurged on pink clothes, matching mittens and shoes. All out of my money, not money sent by them! She was on my breast for two whole months. Jessy and I did not want her to take the bottle. . . . I miss my daughter, you don't know how much.

Diksha is one of the few to mention the racial difference between surrogates and the babies they bear. But this difference does not reduce the kin claims, and even though the baby "looks Japanese," Diksha thinks of her like her own daughter.

The kin ties forged with the baby and the reinterpretation of the blood tie cannot be dismissed as illiterate women's ignorance of modern technology. The surrogates understand and recognize that they have no genetic connection with the baby, but nonetheless they emphasize the ties they have with the baby because of shared substances—blood and sometimes breast milk. In addition, for Diksha, Divya, and Sharda the basis for making claims on the baby is not just shared substance but the labor of bearing and breast-feeding the child. Shared substance and the labor of gestation not only confer identity to the baby but also become the bases for making legitimate claims on the baby.

The kin ties that the surrogates forge on an everyday basis allow them to negotiate the disciplinary discourses that portray surrogates as "disposable mothers." Unlike the medical portrayal of surrogates as temporary and disposable wombs, the surrogates are able to assert that their relationship with the baby is real and often stronger than the one between the genetic mother and baby. Much as the narratives of the women in chapter 7 cannot be classified as merely "remedial work," it would be woefully inadequate to identify these claims to kin ties as mere negotiation strategies. These claims do more than subvert the disciplinary classification of surrogates as disposable mothers; they simultaneously challenge hegemonic bases for making kinship claims. In the kinship claims of these surrogates, shared substance and the *labor* of pregnancy trump not only the mother-child tie based solely on genes but also the semen and blood tie between the father and the child.

"THERE IS NO ROLE OF THE PENIS HERE. NOW IT'S ONLY INJECTIONS!": RECASTING PATRILINEAL TIES

Feminist writers have long recognized and criticized the gendered nature of new reproductive technologies, emphasizing the use and misuse of women's bodies to meet patriarchal ends—the male need to establish the genetic tie. New reproductive technologies are assumed to privilege men's genetic desires and objectify women's procreative capacities. Surrogacy arrangements, in particular, "devalue the mother's relationship to the child in order to exalt the father's" (Roberts 1997, 249). The surrogates at Armaan, however, have a different take on the significance of the genetic tie and the role of men in the surrogacy process.

The surrogacy contract prohibits surrogates from having sexual relations with their husbands. The surrogates living in surrogacy hostels are under additional surveillance and have minimal contact with their husbands. Rita, a surrogate for the second time in two years, jokes about the "emasculation" of husbands through the surrogacy process:

> During my first surrogacy pregnancy, for nine months I was not allowed to do any heavy or risky work. I was not allowed to have any relation [sex] with my husband. [She laughs.] In no other circumstance would he have agreed on that but he needed the money desperately so he had to give in! I am not surprised this thing [surrogacy] is so rare. Tell me, which man will be happy in a situation like this? [Giggling] I am big, but it's not through him. To add to that injury, when I am at the hostel, he has to look after the children and even cook sometimes.

Later in the conversation, Rita talks more about the irrelevant role of the other man—the intended father. "It's hard even for Patelbhai [the genetic father]. He did not even touch me, actually he hasn't even spoken to me. At least Smitadidi [the genetic mother] has seen how I live, what I do. I tell her what the baby is doing inside. She has felt it kicking. Patelbhai is a stranger for me and I am a stranger for him. And yet I am carrying his child."

Rita seems to be arguing that the process of surrogacy requires minimum contribution by the men involved, her husband and the intended father, and is consequently emasculating for them. Previous ethnographies of surrogacy indicate similar narratives used by surrogates in other contexts (Ragone 1994; Teman 2010). In the language of the real women involved in the process, surrogacy is "women's business," with the role of men mostly being sidelined (Teman 2010, 138).

Parvati's narrative reiterates the irrelevant role of men within surrogacy but adds a curious interpretation of the relationship between her husband and the fetus:

My husband stays with his parents nowadays. He visits me sometimes but we usually just talk on phone. We are not supposed to do anything [have sex] for the next few months so why bother? He doesn't *need* to be here. See, with your husband's child there is a constant relation, every night there is a "process" [she makes a gesture with her hands to show penetration] and this makes the seed grow inside the womb. The small seed swells up like this [she mimics a balloon being inflated by a pump] and in nine months is ready to be out. But with surrogacy there is no contact with either your husband or the other male [the biological father] so the child has to be grown by giving me injections.

In Parvati's imagery, her husband's role or the penis's role has been taken over by medicines and technology—an injection, in the case of surrogacy. The injection not only enables procreation but also sustains the pregnancy and effectively replaces the man's role or the penis's role. While Parvati's narrative can be read as an illiterate woman's ignorance of science and biology, the implications of her narratives cannot be trivialized. By de-emphasizing her husband's role in the surrogacy process, Parvati is implicitly reiterating her contribution. Later in the conversation she adds, "I keep some savings aside from the money I get every month [from the couple hiring her] for the month immediately after my delivery. I don't tell my husband about this saving. See, right now I get to eat ice creams, coconut water, milk etc. every day—and they are paying for it. But once the child is out, it is my body [that] will suffer and be weak if I don't continue to eat healthy. I think I deserve it for all I am doing right now."

Regina uses a similar argument to justify her control over the money earned through surrogacy: "Oh no, I haven't talked to my husband about the money or what to do with it. Why would I? I'm the one earning it. If I tell him about it, he'll spend it. Women have to bear so much of sadness for this, why should they give the money to their husbands? *And in any case what does he have to do in this? He did nothing* [emphasis added]. At least the other man gave his sperm, not that that is a very big task either."

In *Recreating Motherhood: Ideology and Technology in a Patriarchal Society* (1989), Barbara Katz Rothman talks about new procreative technologies strengthening the patriarchal ideology of the genetic tie—the patriarchal focus on the seed. "And so we have women, right along with men, saying that what makes a child one's own is the seed, the genetic tie, the 'blood.' And the blood they mean is not the real blood of pregnancy and birth, not the blood of the pulsating cord, the bloody show, the blood of birth, but the metaphorical blood of the genetic tie" (45). The surrogates at Armaan starkly differ from the women in Rothman's imagery: they emphasize the real blood of pregnancy and birth and the sweat of their labor. The male actors involved in surrogacy may have provided the seed, but their kin tie with the baby is undermined because the labor, the effort put in by them in the actual *process* of giving birth is minimal. These kin ties not only challenge patriliny but also allow the women to reiterate their primary role in the surrogacy process and consequently lay claim to at least some of the money earned through surrogacy.

These kin ties that challenge patriliny, however, coexist with other narratives that reinstate the patrilineal and patrilocal focus of kin relations in India. While the emphasis on blood ties based on the substance flow between the baby and the surrogate is a powerful example of creative and dynamic indigenous practices of kinship, they do not completely subvert patriarchal assumptions about relatedness and "ownership." In India, kin ties are often based on the twin notions of patrilineality and patrilocality—descent follows the male line, girls reside with their father before marriage and with husband's kin after marriage and are considered the "property" of first their father and then their husband. The surrogates recognize and validate these assumptions.

Jyoti, hired by an Indian couple residing in the United States, reasons that the act of giving the baby away will be painful, but she is prepared for it.

> Of course I'll feel sad while giving her away. But then I'll also have to give up my daughter once she gets married, won't I? She is *paraya dhan* [someone else's property] and so is this one. Our girls just live with us temporarily. Their real home is with their husband and in-laws. We don't have any right over them, even though we are responsible for them. My daughter is my responsibility for 18 years, and then I have to give her up. But I still remain responsible for anything if she does something wrong. At least with this child I won't be responsible once I give her up. She will be her father's headache.

Jyoti compares the act of giving up the surrogate baby to giving away a daughter at marriage. Indian mothers, she argues, are prepared to send daughters away to their "real" home—that of their husband and in-laws—and the surrogate baby would be nothing different.

Hetal, a 35-year-old surrogate for a couple from Jaipur, echoes the same sentiment:

> I don't think it will be hard giving her away. She is, after all, his property. He is investing so much money in her. We give away our daughters at marriage as well, don't we? Right from the day she is born we start preparing to give her away. We think she was never ours but still we do care for her when she is with us. It will be exactly the same. We know the baby is not ours; they are investing so much money, on my food, my medicines. It's their property. But I will love her like my own. That's the least I can do for them.

Hetal labels the surrogate child the genetic father's "property," property that he has invested in and rightfully owns. Hetal vows to love the baby like her own in return for all the money invested in her medicine, food, and living while she was serving as a surrogate. Hetal and Jyoti's narratives reveal a curious pattern: most surrogates change the sex of the unborn child depending on the intention of the narrative. For instance, when surrogates Parvati, Divya, and Sharda establish some form of relatedness with the baby/fetus, they address it as "he." But when the intention is to normalize the act of giving the baby away, surrogates like Hetal and Jyoti talk of "her" as property to be "given away" at marriage.

While the surrogates' experience and interpretation of ties with the baby cannot be seen as a straightforward challenge to either patriliny or patrilocality, they do seem to indicate the multivocality of kinship. On the one hand, the reinterpretation of the blood tie by Divya, Parvati, and Sharda questions the assumption that genes are the sole basis for making claims on the baby. More powerfully, this reinterpretation is a subversion of hegemonic claims that the child is a product of the father's "seed" and inherits the *father's* blood. Surrogates claim the exact opposite: the child is a product of its gestational mother's blood and a fruit of all the labor and effort of gestation, and this confers identity to the child. On the other hand, surrogates like Jyoti and Hetal, by invoking the genetic parents' "investment," reiterate the patrilineal claim that children are father's "property." Finally, by assimilating surrogacy into the model of giving away daughters when they get married, the surrogates are extending their claims to motherhood while at the same time acknowledging patrilocality.

The surrogates forge kin ties with the baby and lay claims on it by emphasizing the labor of gestation and the effort of giving birth. The second instance of labor in the ties forged by surrogates is the kin labor required to maintain relationships between the intended mother and the gestational mother.

"I KNOW SHE IS YOUNGER THAN I AM, BUT I CALL HER *DIDI*" [ELDER SISTER]: LABORED TIES ACROSS BORDERS

In the early literature on kin relations in North India, kinship often appeared as a bounded sphere closely structured by not just patrilineality (lineage organized around descent in the male line) and patrilocality (residence with husband's kin group), but also caste endogamy (Inden and Nicholas 1977; Madan 1981 Trautmann 1981). North Indian kinship was often portrayed as immutable connections and caste-based exclusion (Carsten 2000). Other scholars, especially anthropologists and ethnographers, have provided powerful criticisms of such "univocal understanding[s] of culture," which are often based on "textual analyses and esoteric rituals" (Dube 1986; Jeffery, Jeffery, and Lyons 1989; Raheja and Gold 1994; Sax 1991; Vatuk 1975). The limitation of such rigid models is that "they can characterize only a very confined sphere of social relations while excluding most of everyday life and everyday interactions that occur beyond these groups" (Lambert 2000, 89). Kinship bonds are not simply an enactment of unambiguous cultural codes but are experienced as ambiguous and fluid, and hence need to be reconstructed, "renewed, and kept viable through a myriad of reciprocities": nurturance, labor, ceremonial participation, shared locality, and simply company (Bodenhorn 2000). It is the *labor* of being related rather than biology that "marks out the kinship sphere from the potentially infinite universe of relatives who may or may not belong" (143).

The surrogates, living in hiding, away from their home, have little opportunity to draw emotional support from their own families. Much like the kin ties forged with the baby, the ties with the intended mother become central to their thinking about surrogacy. As mentioned in chapter 7, these ties allow the surrogate not just to cope with the emotional isolation but also to challenge the medical construction of their relationships as merely contractual and easily disposable. Parvati highlights the labor of maintaining kin ties within surrogacy and talks wistfully about her relationship with the genetic mother. Parvati seems to be confusing what she hopes will happen in the future with reality. Although she has not delivered the baby yet, she speaks about the important role she plays in the baby's life as if it has already happened:

> My couple [intended parents] keep such good relations with me. After delivery, Nandini *didi* [the genetic mother] brought him [the baby] over to me and let me breast-feed him. She sends me invitations for his birthdays. She called me when he got married. When he gets fever she calls and says "Don't worry just pray to God. If you want to see him we'll come and show him to you." I am so lucky to have a sister like her taking care of me. I see how the rest of the surrogates in the clinic get treated.

Curiously, although Parvati calls her relationship with the genetic mother "just like between sisters," she recognizes the status difference. Most surrogates echo Paravati's claim that the relationship was like between sisters, but simultaneously recognized the power difference. The inevitable narrative is "She calls me *didi* [sister] and I call her *barhi didi* [elder sister]", where the hiring sister is referred to as the "elder" and the hired one is "younger'" Parvati explains, "I know Nandini didi [the genetic mother] is younger than I am but I prefer calling her *didi* [elder sister]. She used to call me *didi* as well. But it felt strange because she is from a foreign land, so educated, so well dressed."

In Parvati's case the kin labor performed by her *didi*, which includes allowing her to breast-feed the baby and sending her letters and invitations to the baby's birthdays, is merely fictive. But some of these ties are actually sustained, sometimes even across borders. This is the case for two of the surrogates, Divya and Diksha.

Divya, a former surrogate, emphasizes the continued effort made by Anne, the genetic mother from the United States, to maintain a relationship even after delivery. Perhaps because of her relatively higher education and better economic status, Divya is also one of the few to explicitly talk about reciprocity in their relationship: "Anne came in on the eighth month and for two months she stayed with me. We lived together like a family. My husband got her passport fixed from the American Consulate. We have been in constant touch even after they left. See, she brought me these earrings this time." [She shows me her diamond and white gold earrings.]

Although the surrogates recognize the immense class difference between the intended parents and themselves, they sometimes construct relations in their narratives or fantasies that transcend transnational and class differences. This is reflected in Parvati's fantasy that the couple will continue to treat her like someone special and she will participate in all the important ceremonies, such as the child's birthdays and marriage, like any other family member. Divya believes that she has built a long-lasting friendship with the couple and has become part of a transnational family.

Diksha is a repeat surrogate and, like Divya, she believes her relationship with her first client from Japan is based on mutual respect and reciprocity. Diksha reminisces about the intended mother, Jessy:

> Jessy came to visit me during the *godh bharai* ritual [baby shower organized by the hostel matron for all surrogates], showered me with gifts and gifted Rs 1500 [$30] for my children. It's been three years and today she [the baby born out of surrogacy] would have been three years old. I wished Jessy in the morning on computer and they sent me pictures. You know, they paid me Rupees 1.5 lakhs [$3,000] extra out of happiness and gifted me a laptop when they came to take the baby. Now I can e-mail them using that laptop and they send me pictures by e-mail.

But the kin labor done to maintain this relationship is not based just on material gifts. Diksha recalls the day the clients came to fetch the baby: "When Jessy came and took the baby in her arms, she started crying out of happiness. And you won't believe it, but she kept pointing me [out] to the baby and saying, 'See, this is your mom.' I know the baby did not understand what she was saying to her but it meant a lot to me. So many clients say, 'This is your auntie.' But Jessy said, 'This is your mom.'"

Jessy's symbolic gesture of calling Diksha "mom" and not the more distant "auntie" is an instance of reciprocated kin labor performed by the intended mothers. I discuss the notion of reciprocated kin labor versus "wasted" kin labor in the conclusion. While the relationship between Divya and Anne and Diksha and Jessy are rare examples of ties that cross boundaries of race and nation, there are numerous examples of this tie across caste and religion. Such ties become exceptionally powerful in this region, given the communal tensions witnessed here recently. I confess to Salma, a Muslim surrogate, that I am surprised by her intimate relationship with the intended mother, Preeti, a Hindu non-resident Indian from South Africa. Salma responds by giving me a lecture on politics and religion in India:

Why are you surprised? There is no Hindu-Muslim disharmony amongst the common people. This has been created by the politicians. All their brain is in their *kursi* [throne]. They are making profits and giving us a bad name. Look at Preeti *didi*. She is not a Muslim yet she wanted to keep *roza* [fast that Muslims keep during their festive season] on my behalf because I can't keep it when I am pregnant. Our relationship is not depended on our beliefs. We feel a much stronger bond. Sisters don't need to be from the same mother, right? We are like sisters—just one Muslim and one Christian. I think she is Christian. I haven't asked. But I know she is not from India.

Salma gives more sanctity to her kin ties with the genetic mother than to the bounded sphere prescribed by caste and religious endogamy. The ties of sisterhood between the two women seem to be based on the labor and effort made by the women to maintain these ties: for instance the Hindu genetic mother following a Muslim ritual to bond with her sister. Ironically, when I start a similar conversation with genetic mother Preeti, she confesses that she was, in fact, searching for a high-caste Hindu surrogate but none was available.

I was actually looking for someone who is a Hindu—from a good culture and preferably a Brahman [upper-caste Hindu]. Hasn't it scientifically been proven that what a woman does when she is pregnant affects the child? So if a surrogate does *pooja* [Hindu form of prayer] when she is pregnant, the baby can hear her and be blessed by the prayer. But at that time no other surrogate, except Salma, was available. Even though Salma is a Muslim, I am glad we decided to start this relationship. Now we have become like sisters. No, actually she is more than a sister for me. Not even a sister would do what she is doing for me.

Khanderia has her own explanation for these often reluctant cross-caste and cross-religion connections:

See, the couples can't afford to be picky. At the moment the demand for surrogates is greater than the supply and I think it will remain that way. There are more than 300 intended parents in the waiting list. Only one or two couples have said they are not happy with the surrogate we have given them—the way she looks or her caste and religion. Our philosophy is "take what you get" and if you don't like what you are getting, [she shrugs] too bad for you. And once the two women involved start interacting, they usually form a very strong bond. Some of our international clients stay in touch with the surrogate long after the delivery.

Khanderia believes that the intended parents are forced to "take what they get" since the supply of surrogates is less than the demand for them. Despite the doctor's apparent indifference to the relationships and her commercial interpretation of the relationships emerging out of surrogacy, the surrogates continue to believe in the sanctity of the bonds they form with the intended mothers. Surrogate mother Divya surmises: "Our relationship is made in heaven and we both would do anything to make sure it stays that way."

"WE ALL ARE LIKE FISHES IN A DIRTY POND. WHY LET THE CROCODILE TAKE CONTROL?": SURROGACY HOSTELS AND SURROGATE SISTERS

As discussed in chapter 4, surrogates typically have two kinds of living arrangements: living in the dormitory attached to the clinic directly under Khanderia's care or living in the surrogacy hostel financed by the clinic and run by hostel matron Divya. Ironically these hostels, assumed to be the most concrete manifestation of control, become a powerful site for forming alliances. These gendered spaces, where women live together for the entire length of their pregnancies, generate emotional links and sisterhood among the women. The kin ties between the surrogates, based on shared company and shared residence, often cross boundaries of religion and caste.

Sabina, hired by a couple from Florida and now eight months pregnant, yearns to return to Divya's hostel after her delivery. She wants to spend more time with her "sisters" there—surrogates Mansi and Mona. "If I go back home I'll have to start work immediately. I would rather rest at the hostel for the next two months and spend a few more days with my sisters there. Mansi and Mona and I have become very close. Mansi is very naïve and Mona a bully! So we three make the perfect group."

Despite the surveillance and restrictions, Sabina thinks of the hostel as a "home" where all the pregnant sisters live together and celebrate the different religious festivals.

Divya *didi*'s hostel does not seem like a hostel—it's more like a home to all of us. You know she even has a *godh bharai* function [a Hindu ritual similar to a baby shower]—we get to eat so many sweets and even get our photographs taken. Well, I know we Muslims do not have that ritual but here we all live like family and enjoy all functions. I even celebrated Navratra [a Hindu festival that involves fasting, feasting, and traditional dancing *dandia*] this October and Divya *didi* allowed us to go out and dance *dandia* one night.

Like Sabina, surrogate Mona cherishes the shared meals, rituals, and festivities, but she also mentions the training classes the surrogates attend at the hostel:

We cook our favorite meals together in the kitchen sometimes. Divya *didi* has a cook, but we like cooking with our own hands once in a while. It makes it more like home. My sons visit only once a month but Mansi's children visit more often so I like making small sweets for them.

We all pray together in the evenings in the prayer room; even the Christians join us [the Hindus]. It is not like praying really, more like our evening activity that we all do together, like our English classes. You should come for our class today, we are learning how to answer questions that foreign couples usually ask. [Mansi and Mona laugh and chant together.] What is your name? How many children do you have?

The surrogates live, pray, and eat together for the entire duration of their pregnancies. They even engage in group activities like the evening English and computer classes arranged by the clinic. According to Mona and Sabina, the shared space and shared pain lead to lasting bonds of sisterhood. But not all stories are that of "happy" collective sisterhood. Surrogates often share information about the final payments, and this leads to rivalry and competition. Tina, hired by an Indian settled in Dubai, complains about the informal payment structure where some surrogates, usually the ones assigned to foreigners, get paid much more than the ones hired by "stingy Indians":

> If we are just the womb providers, why are we paid different rates? Doctor Madam usually assigns the "foreigners" to the neediest surrogate. Say, your son has tuberculosis, or your husband has a kidney problem. She makes sure you get a foreign client who pays you at least Rupees 2 lakhs [$5,000]. But needs are relative—I may not have a sick husband but I have starving children. Why should I get stuck with a stingy Indian family? Look at this Puja—she has reserved the next foreigner couple for herself by learning some English. She is very shrewd.

"Shrewd" Puja, the topic of much gossip among other surrogates, accepts that she is competitive. She is one of the few to shun all kin ties with other surrogates. She declares that she is at the clinic to make money and not relationships. She believes the other surrogates envy her because she is a better candidate for surrogacy. "I know Divya and her surrogates talk bad about me. But I am not here to be like them. I want to earn enough to build a house, educate my daughters, and give them a better life. I make sure my couple [the intended parents] is happy with me. I don't care about the rest of them here."

Ramya is another surrogate who is not part of the surrogacy "sisterhood." Other surrogates referred to her as the "money-minded one" because she allegedly managed to negotiate a higher fee. Ramya is often the only surrogate eating her lunch alone in one corner. In all her conversations with me, she actively distances herself from the rest by emphasizing either her upper caste or the relative economic well-being of her extended family:

> You know I am a Brahman and everyone else in my family is very well "settled." Some are in America, some are rich businessmen. If they wanted they could get us "settled" in just one day. But I don't want to ask them. I prefer to just do this. It was easy for me to get a client to hire me and

make them pay me Rs 10,000 ($200) more. I think my fair skin impressed them. Compared to the rest of these dark-skinned girls, I look like a foreigner! I am not like the rest—doing it to build a house or to buy land [she waves her hand at the other surrogates]. And I am not here to make friends. These girls have seen nothing better. But I have seen better days. I don't want any connections to this place. I'll make my money and leave.

During one of our lunches together, Rita explains why Ramya is not part of their lunch group: "We have nothing against her. But she doesn't even tell us her real name. We are all in the same thing and we all have worries. But she treats this like a hospital and nothing else. She is also very money-minded. She doesn't make any effort to join us for lunches or teas. My sister Munni [another surrogate] tried to talk to her one day. She was crying all alone in front of the TV, so Munni tried to make her talk. Talking to others helps, you know. But she refused."

The kin ties are not automatically extended to every surrogate. Ramya and Puja are excluded because they make no effort to engage in kin labor by reciprocating and sharing everyday anxieties with the other surrogates. But that is not the only reason. Both of them are also criticized for being excessively "money-minded," individualistic, and competitive, for treating surrogacy like a contract and the hostel like an institution. In a context where the disciplinary discourses of the clinic as well as the discursive strategies of the surrogates themselves seek to conceal the commercial aspect of surrogacy, Puja and Ramya become deviants.

For most surrogates, however, the hostel is the only community for nine months. The intensive contact allows the surrogates to share information and grievances with each other and sometimes to come up with collective action and even strategies for future employment. Mansi says about her relationship with other surrogates in the hostel: "We are seven surrogates in this room—seven sisters pregnant at the same time! Our villages are not very far—I am sure we will be able to meet each other even after we leave this place. We have convinced Divya didi [the matron] to train us in the beauty business. I don't think English and computer will get us a job, but we may be able to work in a beauty parlor. Once we are done here I want to start a beauty parlor with surrogate Mona."

The kin ties between the surrogates serve as resources and networks for future employment. These ties also serve as a powerful tool against the brokers whom they referred to as kanjoos devrani or the stingy sister-in-law. The "in-law" label, in contrast with ties of sisterhood, is an attempt to dilute any kin ties with brokers and reiterate the business aspect of their relation. The broker-surrogate tie is different and distant from the ties of sisterhood because it is purely commercial and not based on reciprocity. The ties of sisterhood, in turn, become useful in lobbying against the tyranny of the greedy sister-in-law.

Varsha, another resident of the clinic, is a 38-year-old surrogate for a couple from Uttar Pradesh. She starts talking about broker Vimla at the lunch table and all the other surrogates join in: "I was brought here by my *devrani* [sister-in-law] Vimla. Oh, you haven't met her yet? She is the one who gets all of us here. She goes from house to house, knocks on the door and whoever she sees first she grabs them and asks 'Do you want to be a surrogate?' [They all laugh.] No but maybe I shouldn't be telling you about her. I don't want any trouble. Why live in a pond and make the crocodile your enemy?"

While Varsha is reluctant to complain about broker Vimla and "make the crocodile in the pond" her enemy, Regina is defiant. She interrupts Varsha and argues:

Why not? We all are like fishes in a dirty pond. Why let the crocodile take control? I am going to tell her everything. This Vimla, she takes Rs. 10,000 [$200] from us for getting us to the clinic. We take all the pain and she earns so much money. See, we come here because we are desperate but she has made a business out of this. This shouldn't be allowed to happen. We have complained to [the] hostel matron. We want to make sure this is laid out in the contract that no surrogate has to suffer like we did. The couple hiring us should pay extra for people like Vimla *didi*. This money means a lot to us, our children. Why should we have to give it to someone who is not even our relation?

By sticking together "like fishes in a dirty pond," the surrogates develop a sense of collective identity, the ability to demand some minimum rights and protection from exploitation by the brokers. By the time I left the field in 2007, Divya (the hostel matron) had passed the surrogates' message to the Doctor and a special clause had been added to the contract—the intended parents would be responsible for paying any broker involved in the surrogacy process. By 2011, the hostels had started offering two additional vocational courses—beautician training and embroidery training—which are professional skills that the surrogates believe to be more useful than English or computer classes.

SHARED SUBSTANCE, SHARED COMPANY, AND KIN LABOR

Undeniably, commercial surrogacy challenges mainstream assumptions and conceptions of family, kinship, and motherhood. Giving birth to a child in exchange for money and giving that child up right after birth defies the hegemonic model of motherhood, whereby the birth mother commits to be a permanent social mother (Teman 2006, 6). Given these disruptions, it is not surprising that commercial surrogacy provides adequate fodder for exploring new challenges to traditional conceptions of family and kinship. In this chapter I analyzed how real actors negotiate these new challenges to kinship and motherhood. As commercial surrogates in India, the women not only negotiate the usual anomalies that the process of surrogacy entails, but also circumstances specific to surrogacy in India—namely, living with other surrogates during the months of pregnancy, having limited contact with their own families during the pregnancy, and delivering babies for people from different classes, castes, religions, and even different races and nations. The surrogates negotiate these challenges by constructing new bases for kinship. In their daily lives, shared substance, shared company, the labor of gestation and giving birth, as well as the continuous labor required to maintain kin relationships, replace procreation as the primary determinants of kin ties.

What implications do these everyday forms of kinship, based on labor and substance, have for existing conceptualizations of kinship? The surrogates' lived experience of kinship and fluid construction of substance challenge existing work on kinship on three major grounds. First, the surrogates' narratives offer an alternative interpretation of the blood tie—a tie based on substance rather than one based solely on nature or biology. Second and simultaneously, these ties override the contributions made by men, making space for a more complex interpretation of patriliny and patrilocality than is indicated by existing theories on Indian kinship. The gestational mother can make claims on the baby not just because her blood nourishes the fetus but also because she is *entitled* to it. It is a fruit of all the effort she has put in, the labor of gestation and of giving birth. Men become irrelevant to the process, as their contribution to the "labor" of procreation is minimal. In her pioneering work, cultural anthropologist Micaela di Leonardo (1987) introduced the concept of "kin work" to refer to the "conception, maintenance, and ritual celebration of cross-household kin ties" (442). Revealing the actual labor embodied in what we culturally conceive as love and considering the political uses of this labor help to denaturalize kin ties and highlight the gendered forms of labor inherent in forming and maintaining kin ties. The surrogates' constructions of kinship denaturalize kin ties by highlighting *labor* as a basis for making kinship claims. This includes not just the labor of gestation and giving birth but also the effort put in by the surrogates and intended mothers of sending gifts, writing letters, and keeping in touch with each other even after the delivery of the baby. It also includes the work done by the surrogates to reciprocate a feeling of community by sharing space, food, rituals, and everyday anxieties with one another. Third and finally, these kin ties forged with intended mothers and other surrogates cross borders of class, religion, and sometimes race and nation. They disrupt the construction of Indian kinship as a bounded sphere constrained by not just patriliny but also interactions within the same caste and religion. For daily existence and negotiations, shared company, continuous labor, and the effort of reciprocities take precedence over formal and restrictive models of interactions, and ties of "sisterhood" seemingly cross all borders in Garv.

It would be facile to end this chapter without acknowledging the irony of these kin ties. The surrogates form kin ties that disrupt the sanctity of biology and genes within a system that might well be the pinnacle of the commodification of the genetic tie. The high demand for gestational surrogacy occurs precisely because the genetic tie remains a powerful and enduring basis of human attachment. People are ready to travel halfway across the world and hire an Indian surrogate to fulfill their yearning to share a genetic tie with their children. The perceived beauty of gestational surrogacy, relative to traditional surrogacy or transnational adoption, is that the hiring couple need *not* cross any borders; the child born will carry its parents' genes and subsequently their race, caste, and religion. For ironically, in the end, the surrogate's claims on the baby don't prevent it from being taken away from her—very often, immediately after birth.

The everyday and creative kin ties established by the surrogates may pose very little threat to the fundamental (genetic) foundation of kinship. But these ties represent a constant process of renegotiation of the bases for forming ties at the local level. They demonstrate the ability of a group of women to reiterate the role of shared substance and kin labor in forming and maintaining kin ties and to use these claims to their own advantage. The small, seemingly trivial claims made by the women in this study provoke a reappraisal of existing assumptions surrounding kinship. Unlike classic kinship models, these new forms of kinship seem to be open to manipulations and transformations. They offer new possibilities for understanding how relatedness may be composed of various components—shared substance, shared company, and the labor of women.

9 ✆ CONCLUSION

APORIA OF SURROGACY

WHEN I started the research for this book in 2006, commercial surrogacy was a rare occurrence in India. Most fertility clinics steered clear of surrogacy or required that the clients arrange for their own surrogate. The international publicity and the "success" of Armaan Maternity Clinic started a trend, and by 2013 there were clinics offering surrogacy services in almost every city in India. This book explores the workings of this new labor market for wombs and analyzes the experiences of the laborers as they negotiate the peculiarities of this market—where production and reproduction literally merge. As one can imagine, a market in wombs is not a simple one. In this concluding section, I raise some critical questions for demystifying the aporia of surrogacy.

A fundamentally paradoxical characteristic of commercial surrogacy resonates with other gendered forms of labor like domestic work and sex work. On the one hand, commercial surrogacy becomes a powerful challenge to the age-old dichotomy constructed between production and reproduction. Women's reproductive capacities are valued and monetized outside of the so-called private sphere. As surrogates, women use their bodies, wombs and sometimes breasts, as instruments of labor. But just as commercial surrogacy subverts these gendered dichotomies, it simultaneously reifies them. When reproducing bodies of women become the only source, requirement, and product of a labor market, and fertility becomes the only asset women can use to earn wages, women essentially get reduced to their reproductive capacity, ultimately reifying their historically constructed role in the gender division of labor. The second paradox revealed in the book is specific to the Indian context, where a labor market in assisted conception is booming in a country with a historically aggressive anti-natalist agenda. The fertility of lower-class women in India has previously been constructed as not just undesirable at individual levels but a social danger. In the context of surrogacy, this fertility gets temporarily revalued as lower-class women become reproducers for clients who are relatively more privileged. This book argues that such a practice is not simply a glaring example of stratified reproduction but a product of conscious state policies and a neoliberal eugenic imperative. The stratified reproduction in India, surrogacy being one of its manifestations, is a result of intentional state priorities and an inevitable consequence of the present global division of both productive and reproductive labor.

It becomes even more critical to emphasize these contradictions because they do not merely engage feminist debates and state policies. They have real-life consequences at the everyday level: they shape the disciplinary project devised to manufacture a perfect surrogate and the discursive tools employed by the surrogates to resist that project. The book reveals that the dual mother-worker identity is strategically used by the clinic as a repressive and effective tool of discipline and control. At various stages of the disciplinary process, the clinic employs the rhetoric of "good motherhood" to restrain the surrogates as workers, and the rhetoric of "good workerhood" to contain them as mothers. While a good worker is professional, a good mother-worker is expected to treat the fetus growing inside her as her own, not to be business-minded, and to refrain from negotiating the wages involved. Thus during the contract period and the period of pregnancy, a surrogate's motherhood is expected to take primacy and a surrogate who demands a wage increase is stigmatized as a dirty prostitute. But while a good mother loves her child unconditionally and forever, the disciplinary project requires a good mother-worker to love the child only temporarily. On delivery, her workerhood should take primacy, so that she becomes the good contract worker who adheres to the contract and gives up the baby willingly. Ultimately, through a strategic use of the dual mother-worker identity, the clinic constructs the perfect mother-worker of the clients' dream.

Surrogates, however, are not simply constructs of disciplinary power and discourse. The resistive strategies of the surrogates, in essence, explicate the complex web of power relations. At various stages of the surrogacy process, the surrogates negotiate with their family and the clinic to gain control over their own bodies and reproductive futures. Although these negotiations are ostensibly at the micro-political level, often a response to the disciplinary tactics used by the clinic and a response to the medical construction of surrogates as dirty workers and disposable mothers, they are affected by and have repercussions at the macro level, namely at the level of the state. Simultaneously, they often speak to the unequal power relationships between the buyers and sellers of surrogacy, inequalities based on race, class, and citizenship.

The first arena for individual resistance takes the form of discursive resistances—individual attempts to negotiate the various disciplinary discourses employed by the clinic, the media, and the community through the strategic use of alternative narrative and speech. Surrogates resist the construction of surrogates as "disposable and dirty workers" and as "disposable mothers." In sharp contrast to the surrogate-prostitute analogy used by the clinic and the media, the surrogates construct themselves as moral and needy mothers. While on the one hand, these alternative constructions of surrogacy by the surrogates affirm their dignity and sense of self-worth, on the other hand, they replicate certain gender hierarchies. Ironically, while the focus of this study has been on surrogacy as labor, most surrogates do not speak of surrogacy as paid work or work that they have chosen. It is almost as if the surrogates do not resist the image of women as selfless dutiful mothers whose primary role is to serve the family. Similarly, the vigorous defense of their husbands' moral worth within these narratives of morality indicates that the women are overcompensating for their (temporary) role as breadwinners.

Wombs in Labor analyzes another powerful instance of individual resistance as well—surrogates challenge the medical construction of surrogates as disposable mothers by forging kin ties with the baby and the intended mothers. Surrogates' constructions of kinship denaturalize kin ties by highlighting *labor* and not genes or patriliny as a basis for making kinship claims. Moreover, the ties with intended mothers from all over the world disrupt the construction of Indian kinship as a bounded endogamous sphere constrained by race, caste, and religion. But as with other instances of discursive and individual resistances analyzed in the book, this too has contradictory impacts. As the surrogates emphasize the special ties with the baby and the intended mother, they undermine their identity as wage-earning laborers and further erode their ability to negotiate wages. Simultaneously, the portrayal of the intended mother (from a wealthier nation) as someone who would rescue the surrogate from desperate poverty brings in issues of new forms of subjection based on race and class domination.

The bodies of the surrogates are the third arena of individual resistance. Here too the contradictory impact of individual resistance is evident. The surrogates resist instructions of the state, their husbands, and their families by postponing sterilization and other reproductive decisions in order to use their bodies for labor. At the micro-political level, these negotiations with the family are victories for women's self-esteem, giving them the ability to maneuver in their families, and make money using the only resource they really have—their bodies. As the surrogates use their bodies for "productive" ends, they subvert the anti-natalist state portrayal of the bodies of poor women as "wasteful." But *Wombs in Labor* reveals the irony of this embodied resistance—as these women align their own reproduction to meet the needs of commercial surrogacy, as they undergo abortions and forgo having their own children, they end up conforming to the state imperative of selective anti-natalism.

The last arena for resistance explored in this book is the physical space of the surrogacy hostels and the ties and networks formed by the surrogates within that space. Oddly enough, the gendered space of the surrogacy hostel, typically imagined to be the most repressive form of surveillance, becomes an avenue for collective resistance. Some women use the hostel space to share information and grievances. Others come up with acts of collective action and even strategies for future employment. By the time I left the field, the surrogates had collectively asked for some vital changes in the contract to reduce exploitation by brokers. A few surrogates manage to sustain these kin ties even after delivery. In the epilogue I describe one such instance in more detail—where two surrogates develop the kin ties forged within the hostel space into a business partnership.

In her book *Living the Body: Embodiment, Womanhood, and Identity in Contemporary India* (2009), Meenakshi Thapan finds recourse in Derrida's theory of aporias in order to understand the "dual characteristic of resistance, symbolizing both agency and loss, subversion and reification." This dual characteristic, Thapan argues, does not suggest the "eventual voicelessness and despair of the gendered subject but a state of being in an impasse, which allows the impossible movement of traversing—without crossing—the ultimate border" (Thapan 2009, 164). For Thapan, and other scholars of everyday resistances, it becomes imperative just to acknowledge women's efforts at resistance. These attempts indicate not only their awareness of their condition but also a constant struggle to negotiate it to their advantage, even if not to overcome it. It is in "the moment of resistance" that "the possibility of openness and change" exists (171). In this book, the puzzling dual nature or the aporias of resistance complicate notions of domination and subversion. But the dual nature of resistances brings attention back to the peculiarity of this new form of labor—labor that lies on the cusp of production and reproduction. The acts of resistance by the surrogates sometimes subvert but often reify assumptions about what it means to be a surrogate mother. But just as importantly, by challenging the dichotomy between production and reproduction, they also disrupt assumptions about what it means to be a mother and a worker. These disruptions, albeit with paradoxical consequences, shape women's identities as laborers, as mothers, and as compatriots in a stigmatized and marginalized labor option.

It is likely that the everyday resistances by the surrogates that I highlight in this book pose very little threat to the fundamentally exploitative structure of transnational surrogacy. What they do represent, however, is a constant process of negotiation and strategizing at the local level. While these forms of resistance are aimed at disciplinary discourses and practices, they sometimes transform women's sense of individual and collective identity as well, and disrupt their place in the household, workplace, and community. They provoke a reappraisal of existing assumptions surrounding not just surrogacy but our understanding of new forms of women's labor, new bases for forming kin ties, and novel responses to new reproductive technologies and biomedicalization.

FROM MORALS TO LAWS

The ambiguity and stigma surrounding labor markets like commercial surrogacy (and, for that matter, sex work) reflect anxieties about women trespassing the boundaries between non-market and market, and between reproduction and production. These anxieties are so deeply entrenched in the working of these markets that it is impossible to locate labor as something entirely divorced from issues of morality. In various sections of this study I explored the creative ways in which women negotiate the relationship between this new form of labor and morality. These strategies range from attempts to engage in boundary work, emphasizing their higher motivations in becoming a surrogate, resorting to divinity, to claiming kin ties with the baby and the clients. These anxieties inevitably seeped into my fieldwork and research. People are often disturbed by my apparent "objective" stance and repeatedly ask questions like "What is *your* personal opinion of commercial surrogacy in India?" "Do you think it is right or wrong?" "Do you think the Doctor is evil?" My responses to such questions have varied from acute ambivalence to determined unambiguity. On the one hand, I am convinced that there is nothing *inherently* immoral about surrogacy. On the other hand, I feel uncomfortable with the assumption that since I posit surrogacy as labor, I want India to develop a flourishing business in the outsourcing of wombs. In the concluding section of this study, I broaden the debate by evaluating some of the anxieties regarding surrogacy in general as well as concerns specific to the form commercial surrogacy takes in India. At the same time I speculate about the implications of these anxieties for future policies and laws.

The lens through which we view surrogacy will shape the ultimate policies and regulations devised. If we use the lens of morality, we might well come to the conclusion that commercial surrogacy is inherently immoral and undesirable. It defies laws of nature, family, and religion and is a commercialization of motherhood, of the act of giving birth, and of children. An obvious policy corollary for a class of action considered intrinsically wrong is to prohibit it by imposing a formal ban. I have already expressed my discomfort with the "inherent immorality" claim, especially since it reifies the dichotomy between production and reproduction, and universalizes and naturalizes the so-called "sacred" bond between mother and child. But even if we step out of the morality box, we can still argue that surrogacy is undesirable, and more specifically that it is undesirable in the *Indian* context. The argument could be that in a country where most people cannot afford even basic health care, investment in ART diverts essential resources to relatively less urgent needs. One can reasonably question the desirability of investment in ART like surrogacy when only 8 percent to 10 percent of the Indian population suffers from infertility, and nearly 98 percent of that is secondary infertility caused by infections, malnutrition, questionable contraceptive use, and inadequate prenatal and postnatal care (Qadeer 2010a). Strengthening primary healthcare services to ensure good prenatal, postnatal, and childbirth services, and thus avoid many obstetric and gynecological problems, should be a state priority rather than investment in ART that most cannot afford.

Secondly, ART and surrogacy may be undesirable in India given the specific cultural context of son preference. The last decade has highlighted the growing (mis)use of ART for sex selection; for instance, genetic manipulation at the pre-implantation stage (manipulation to ensure a male offspring) has been reported from many parts of India.[1] While a law passed in 1996 bans the use of prenatal genetic diagnostic techniques (such as amniocentesis) to determine fetal sex, there is no law regarding pre-implantation genetic diagnosis and genetic engineering. Doctors and IVF clinics in India have countered all criticism of these sex-selection procedures by resorting to the predictable language of choice and by using the less controversial label "family balancing" (Malpani, Malpani, and Modi 2002). But when technology changes faster than mind-sets, ART can become treacherous (Unnithan-Kumar 2010). Finally, it can be argued that *transnational* surrogacy in India is undesirable because of its exceptionally exploitative potential. Transnational surrogacy, in which women in the global south are providing cheap wombs for women in the global north, has relatively more potential for exploitation than within-border surrogacy, or surrogacy in the global north, because of the extreme inequalities in power (based on class, race, and national differences) between the client and the surrogate in India. When intended parents travel from countries in the global north to access services in the global south, there is an additional anxiety that such travel reifies global inequalities by making the bodies (and cells, organs, and tissues) of people in resource-poor countries more "bioavailable" than people in other locales (Cohen 2005; Heng 2007; Pande 2011; Whittaker and Speier 2010). This becomes even more striking for clinics where the presence of surrogacy hostels, surrogacy brokers, and a high level of surveillance of surrogates adds to the potential for exploitation.

How can we address these anxieties surrounding surrogacy in India? There are two possible policy options: an outright ban or a regulatory framework. Whatever our stance on surrogacy, I would caution against an outright ban on surrogacy. People's desire for genetic babies is unlikely to diminish in the near future. Development in relevant assisted reproductive technologies cannot be reversed, and with globalization, clients will continue to cross borders to make use of these technologies. A *national* ban is not just unrealistic but also undesirable. Banning surrogacy in India will just push it underground, further stigmatizing the profession and the women involved and undermining their rights as workers.[2] If there is one thing to be learned from the experience of sex workers, the abolitionist tendency can only be calamitous for working women, whether in sex work or commercial surrogacy. Imposing a comprehensive ban on surrogacy in India will likely simply shift the practice to another country in the global south.

An alternative is to advocate for either a *global* ban on *commercial* surrogacy or a global ban on *cross-border* commercial surrogacy. Several countries have made a case for banning commercial, paid surrogacy but permitting altruistic surrogacy—surrogacy arrangements in which the surrogate is not paid for her services (except reasonable expenses connected with her pregnancy and care) and is motivated mainly by a desire to help an infertile couple to have a child of their own. It has been argued that because altruistic surrogacy excludes commercial elements, it does not commodify children or the reproductive process. Moreover, advocates of altruistic surrogacy claim that non-commercial surrogacy enables us to recognize and appreciate the real value in surrogacy. Much like voluntary blood donation, the practice of altruistic surrogacy allegedly underscores the indispensability of the gestational role and defines surrogacy as "a relationship of mutual understanding and generosity between the surrogate and the infertile couple," rather than just a contractual relationship (Baker 1996, 41). Altruistic surrogacy, however, is not without its critics. One feminist objection to altruistic surrogacy is that it reinforces the stereotype of women as "naturally" nurturant and selfless. For instance, Sharyn R. Anleu (1992) and Janice Raymond (1990) have argued that the distinction between commercial and altruistic surrogacy is "socially constructed" and, in essence, altruistic surrogacy oppresses women under the guise of a "moral celebration" of their altruism.

An alternative is to impose a ban on all *cross-border* surrogacy, since it arguably increases the likelihood of exploitation. Legal scholars and bioethicists, especially in the European Union region, have been debating the costs and benefits of permitting cross-border reproductive travel for services like surrogacy. Some, like bioethicist Guido Pennings, believe that cross-border reproductive travel is an obvious and fair solution to restrictive national legislation. It promotes moral pluralism in democratic states, since it "prevents the frontal clash between the majority who imposes its view and the minority who claim to have a moral right to some medical service" (Pennings 2002). Others, like legal scholars John Robertson (2004) and Robert Storrow (2010), see such travel as not only a poor solution but also counterproductive to moral and political pluralism. It allows only a certain class of people—the ones with the economic means to travel—the option to escape the restraints of the law. Moreover, in effect, the availability of cross-border options allows national governments to enact stricter laws at home than they might otherwise have the political will to enact. Strict national laws, in turn, export the morally contentious industry to some other country, very often to a country in the global south. The increasing clientele of surrogacy clinics in India from countries with national bans on commercial surrogacy (for instance, the U.K., Germany, and Spain) is an indication of this trend. With the rise in cross-border surrogacy, most countries have started recognizing the need to incorporate these new complexities in their policies around surrogacy. Some countries, for instance Turkey and Malaysia, have extended their restrictive approach to cross-border surrogacy and prohibit their citizens from obtaining surrogacy procedures abroad. Others, like France, the U.K., Germany, Spain, and Japan, attempt to discourage their citizens from pursuing surrogacy abroad by withholding legal recognition of such cases (Storrow 2010). Children born out of surrogacy arrangements abroad, for instance, may not be given travel documents or granted citizenship status. With the rise in international legal disputes regarding the citizenship of children born out of surrogacy in India, some countries are contemplating a different strategy—making their *domestic* surrogacy laws less restrictive so that their nationals need not travel outside their borders to access this technology. Iceland, Norway, and Sweden, which currently prohibit all kinds of surrogacy arrangements, are currently debating a shift toward a less restrictive approach that would allow altruistic surrogacy at home to discourage its citizens from going abroad in search of surrogates.

Short of an outright ban on surrogacy, can we develop more-stringent laws to *regulate* national and international surrogacy? Janice Raymond, in a caustic critique of regulatory policies, argued that "regulation functions as quality control rather than as critical challenge. . . . It gives the surrogate brokers, for example, a stable marketing environment and makes the process of surrogacy more convenient for the client and broker" (1993, 207). A "critical challenge," however, needs to be pragmatic rather than idealistic. Given that countries like India will most likely lack the political will to effectively implement a ban on surrogacy, the more likely outcome of a ban would be to make surrogates even more vulnerable, without any protection from brokers and clients. To quote Debora Spar, author of *The Baby Business* (2006): "Unless one posits, however, that the existence of global inequality renders all economic choices moot; and until there is any path by which these inequalities can feasibly be addressed, denying women this particular choice seems oddly counter-productive. It also does not square with the kind of logic applied to other areas of the global labour market . . . where concerns about global inequality lead toward international rules and regulations, not a total prohibition of the activity involved" (305).

THE MATTER OF REGULATION:
"FAIR TRADE SURROGACY"?

The Indian Council of Medical Research (ICMR) made an attempt at regulating the industry when it included some references to surrogacy in the broader National Guidelines for Accreditation, Supervision, and Regulation of Assisted Reproductive Technology (ART) clinics in India in 2005, and in the more recent draft ART Regulatory Bill in 2010. These guidelines remained non-binding. The spate of international legal battles since 2010 over citizenship and custody of children born through surrogacy forced the government to get serious about binding regulations. In 2013 the directorate general of health services (DGHS) stirred up a controversy by suggesting some changes to the clauses in ART bill—that the option of surrogacy be restricted to married, infertile couples of Indian origin. This was a restrictive variant of the 2012 stipulation by the Home Ministry that gay couples, single men and women, and couples from countries where surrogacy is illegal be prohibited from hiring a commercial surrogate in India. In essence, the DGHS proposal, if implemented, would ban foreigners, homosexuals, and people in live-in relationships from having a baby born out of surrogacy in India. Before we dismiss these proposals as "draconian and archaic" or hail them as a pioneering attempt by a state to protect its citizens, let's speculate a little about the reasons for the government's proposing such changes, at the cost of losing a $2 billion industry. The obvious answer: to avoid more international legal battles. The official answer: to better protect the rights of the child and ensure that only people in stable relationships and from countries that agree to give the child citizenship are allowed to have babies through surrogacy.[3] Not surprisingly, the people criticizing these proposals pull out their liberal "right to parenthood" card—everyone should have the right to have a child of their own. I suspect that the camps on both sides of the divide are failing to prioritize a vital part of the story: the rights of the surrogates. The ongoing controversy about the proposed *changes* to clauses in the ART bill also threatens to divert attention from the critical debate about the *existing* clauses in the ART bill. Feminist and health activists have criticized the bill for exactly the reasons I suggest above: that the bill is totally inadequate in addressing the concerns of surrogates as workers, or in protecting their health and well-being. (Qadeer 2009; SAMA 2010). The bill is especially hazy on such critical issues as the rights of the surrogate, details of the contracts, role of different intermediaries, nature of "informed consent," nature of compensation, and legal, medical, and post-partum assistance for the surrogates.

The reality is that surrogacy cannot be resolved as a national issue or by closing borders. Given the nature of this industry, it would be naïve to expect that any national law will be enforced and effective on its own. As Wendy Chavkin (2010) surmises, "With increasing globalization, a country's policy decisions on reproduction are not contained by national borders, as people, products, body parts, technologies and ideas move across borders" (7). A more practical step might be to have an open international dialogue on the nature of this industry. Medical practitioner Casey Humbyrd (2009) proposes a move toward such an international dialogue and regulation in her guide to "fair trade practices" in international surrogacy. Humbyrd provides a provocative argument in favor of "applying Fair Trade principles to international surrogacy" in order to ensure that the benefits of surrogacy "are justly shared between the participating parties" and are beneficial to those who are the "weakest in the supply chain"—the surrogates (Humbyrd 2009, 116).[4] Although Humbyrd fails to address how this regulatory and compensation framework can be implemented, I find it constructive to evaluate and extend some of her policy insights based on my ethnographic findings. For instance, Humbyrd briefly mentions that a "fair price in the regional or local context" is "one that has been agreed through dialogue and participation." She goes on to add that there is a need for "transparency and accountability . . . of financial transactions between surrogacy brokers, prospective parents and surrogate mothers." I extend Humbyrd's insights and propose an international model of surrogacy founded on openness and transparency on three fronts: in the structure of payments, in the medical process, and in the relationships forged within surrogacy.

Transparency in financial transaction and allowing wage settlements through dialogue between the surrogates and the intended parents are valuable recommendations, highlighted by the surrogates themselves. Some clauses in the current bill attempt to address concerns about financial transparency, but these are completely inadequate. Oddly, while the bill seems to promote the "business" of surrogacy and other ART, it is strangely myopic in its understanding of the realities of this industry. Social scientist and community health activist Imrana Qadeer (2010a) has highlighted many instances of this myopia. For instance, the bill pays very little attention to details of administration of the contract between the surrogate and the intended parents. There is little information on how the money transaction would actually take place, and no mechanism to ensure the enforcement of other financial aspects of the contract is proposed in the bill. The bill fails to clearly lay out the details of the financial arrangement between the surrogate and the intended parents. Although it emphasizes the need to have a legally binding contract, it does not clarify whether the intended parents would reimburse all prenatal and postnatal care expenses as well as the opportunity cost of not being able to work after a surgery. It does not require that surrogates be provided legal assistance in case of any conflicts during the surrogacy arrangement. The payment structure reflects that priority is accorded to the intended parents and not to the surrogates. For instance, the latest draft of the bill recommends that payment be made to the surrogate in five installments, with the majority (75 percent) to be paid upon the delivery of the baby (SAMA 2010). This structure clearly disadvantages surrogates, especially in the event of a late miscarriage.

A meaningful discussion on transparency in financial transactions, however, needs to consider the distinctive attributes of this work. For instance, surrogacy involves intense amounts of body work and emotional work and often forges relationships, arguably more intimate ones than that between the buyer and the seller in many other markets. Consequently, national or international laws cannot exclude the potential for change through dialogue and negotiations at the local level. The intimate and personal relationships that surrogates forge with their clients are not just a source of potential exploitation for the worker but can be a basis for negotiating everyday advantages. For instance, scholars have indicated that the personalized employer-employee relationships forged in the provision of reproductive services—often portrayed as disempowering and archaic—are not necessarily perceived as negative by the workers themselves. Workers often perceive these intimate relationships as a way to gain extra benefits.[5] Certain clauses mentioned in the bill seem to indicate that the couple and the surrogate can mutually decide the payment. But given that most surrogates are illiterate and/or have little familiarity with legal contracts, negotiations have to be preceded by counseling and provision of information. If the surrogate is either unable or unwilling to negotiate all the financial details on her own, a social worker or financial counselor could facilitate this process.

For surrogacy in India, transparency in the second arena—medical process—needs to be much more than a signature indicating informed consent. For women who have little experience with biomedical technologies and professional medicine, being "aware" of the medical requirements and implications of ART cannot take the form of a mere signature, but should be a continuous process of explanation and interaction over a period of time. SAMA, a Delhi-based women's health group and one of the few organizations to actively condemn the proposed bill, has highlighted other health-related loopholes in the bill and the obvious biases in favor of clinics and clients (SAMA 2010).[6] For instance, the bill downplays the potential harm the various drugs and procedures can have on the health of surrogates. Moreover, since the assumption is that traditional surrogates, who are genetically connected to the baby, are likely to be more attached to the baby, the bill prohibits surrogates from being the egg donor. In essence, the bill makes sure that to become a surrogate, a woman would have to undergo IVF even if her eggs were viable and she could bear the child through the much simpler process of artificial insemination. Other clauses in the bill further confirm that the needs of the clients are prioritized over the surrogate's physical and emotional well-being. To ensure that the surrogate has no opportunity to change her mind or get attached to the baby, the bill recommends separation of the baby from the surrogate immediately after delivery. To increase the chance of a successful birth, the bill permits five live births to a woman and three cycles of ova transfer per client without any reference to the health risks that this process entails for the surrogate. Even the right to demand abortion and fetal reduction is given to the intended parents, and the surrogate is mandated to comply with these decisions made by others about her body. To ensure maximum benefits of international clients and surveillance of the surrogate pregnancy the bill states that for international couples commissioning a surrogacy, a local guardian will be appointed for the surrogate mother. This "guardian" will presumably play a role similar to that of hostel matrons at Garv and be responsible for supervising the life of the surrogate during the months of pregnancy. The surrogate's right to privacy and physical integrity, however, is given little consideration in the draft bill. There is no mention of "surrogacy hostels" of the kind that are coming up in Garv or any debating on the ethics of a "guardian" or other forms of surveillance. The draft bill ignores one of the primary factors that shape surrogacy in India—the stigma attached to surrogacy and surrogates. This stigma often pushes women into accepting the dormitory-style lifestyle and surveillance of their surrogate pregnancy in hostels. The interests of clients and clinics, however, are fully protected, with all risks transferred to the surrogate—the clinic or the client cannot be held responsible for her death during pregnancy or delivery, or for any complication during fetal reduction.

The final arena where transparency is critical is in the complex layers of social interactions embedded within surrogacy. American anthropologist Paul Rabinow coined the term "biosociality" to capture the "new" kinds of identities, social groupings, and social interactions made possible by developments in genetics (Rabinow 1996). Since then, scholars have extended the concept to explore emerging bonds of community grounded in new biotechnologies—from genome projects to IVF (Gibbon and Novas 2008). For the analytics of biosociality to be relevant for surrogacy we need to pay closer attention to the relationships emerging in and through these markets, relationships that are often abruptly terminated in our pursuit of anonymity and privacy. In his work on what he labels the "red market" or the market in body parts, body fluids, organs, and wombs, journalist Scott Carney (2010) urges us to reevaluate the emphasis on privacy and anonymity in these unusual markets. In the name of preserving the privacy of individuals involved in the supply chain, the providers of essential, emotional, and bodily services are made nameless, faceless, anonymous, and disposable—and buyers can conveniently forget that what is being produced is not just a baby but also relationships.

What if, for once, we abandon our single-minded pursuit of privacy and instead advocate for open acknowledgment of these relationships—an appreciation of the complex and demanding nature of labor provided by each individual surrogate? What if we make visible the gestational and emotional work done by the surrogates (Hochschild 2009)? This call for openness and transparency is not as idealistic as it may sound. Legislation and policies around national and intercountry adoption have long made this a central concern. Studies on the growing industry of surrogacy indicate the urgent need to make productive comparisons between intercountry adoption and transnational surrogacy laws. For instance, social work scholars Karen Smith Rotabi and Nicole Footen Bromfield (2012), who focus primarily on inter-country adoptions and "adoption frauds" in Guatemala, have predicted that surrogacy may well be replacing adoption in countries like Guatemala. They argue that the consistent increase in the global demand for healthy young children, and a decline in adoption opportunities, has resulted in an increase in the "price of young children" as well as an increase in the waiting time for the placement of these children. International surrogacy and in vitro fertilization are emerging as lucrative alternatives. In a more tongue-in-cheek comparison, Anoop

Gupta, an Indian fertility doctor, has surmised, "Surrogacy is the new adoption" (quoted in Twine 2011, 16). Whether surrogacy is indeed the new adoption is debatable, but the "open" model of adoption can provide a guiding framework for future policies (Satz 1992).[7]

An open and transparent model of transnational surrogacy brings into focus another intricacy that has, curiously, escaped much of the discussion—the recognition that the *final "product" of this market is a living child*. Unlike in the case of adoption, where many countries (including India) have ratified the Hague Adoption Convention (1993) and have devised comprehensive laws regarding the rights of the adopted child, the rights of children born through surrogacy become a topic of discussion only during custody disputes.[8] More research is required in the future to gauge the impact of gestation on the lives of children. But for now we can reasonably assume that issues that have been relevant for inter-country adoption will arise in the future for transnational surrogacy as well. For instance, should the child born through surrogacy be told about his or her womb mother in India? Should a child be allowed to contact his or her birth mother? These are just some of the questions that will need answering in a not-so-distant future.

What we decide about this remarkable new form of women's labor and what is decided in the Indian Parliament will undoubtedly shape the future of surrogacy in India. It will also likely impact the future of surrogacy in other parts of the world as well. Already private clinics in Ukraine and Thailand have started advertising their competitive rates and flexible laws. For instance, Thailand has been quick to benefit from India's 2012 government stipulation of restricting surrogacy in India to married heterosexual couples. In addition, Thailand offers something that India cannot legally offer: "the ability to choose your child's sex."[9] Ukraine, meanwhile, has started offering "Euroconsulting," advertised as a "unique package approach to surrogacy" that protects the clients' interests from the moment they sign a contract until they receive the official birth certificate of the child. Just as importantly, the government's decisions will have an impact on the experiences of the women workers. Ramya, a surrogate mother, predicts that women would continue to do this work irrespective of the government's decision. But the law would shape the working conditions and the distribution of profits:

> Women in our country will continue to do this, whether the government likes it or not, whether you like it or not! This is the best option available for many of us. If the government declares this to be a bad thing, we will

do this in hiding, like prisoners, ashamed and weeping over our misfortune. If they declare this "a good thing," we will do it with the support of our family and neighbors, with our children next to us. We still won't sing about it proudly or yell it out to our neighbours, but we will do it with some normalcy . . .

. . . I might not be as educated as you are, but I do understand one thing: too many people gain from this surrogacy. [She counts on her fingers.] My family, Vimla [the broker] and her family, Doctor Madam, the rickshaw puller [*rickshawalla*] outside who carries the intended mother [*didi*] to her hotel, the airline pilot [*airplanewalla*] who brings her from America. Our government must be getting something too. They would not want this to stop. All they will do is decide who gets more and who gets less in this business.

FROM GLOBAL SISTERHOOD TO TRANSNATIONAL FEMINISM

An exclusive dependence on national and international policymakers to initiate a meaningful dialogue is not only naïve but also inappropriate. Is there another space for dialogue, collective consciousness, and collective action? A collective is already in its nascent stage with the front-runners—the surrogates. On my last visit to the clinic I met with a group of six "veteran" surrogates—women who have been involved in this industry for nearly six years. I was curious to hear their reflections on the developments in the industry since its inception. What changes do they see? What changes would they like to see? There was little ambiguity about the first question. There was consensus that there has been a significant, albeit insufficient, increase in payments. Rita succinctly reported:

> It sounds strange, but *the change I like is the payment. And what I would like to change is also the payment* [emphasis added]. See, I got less than 1 lakh [$2,000] for my first [surrogacy]. Right now women get even up to 5 lakh [$10,000]. That is good. But is that enough? What if I want to build a house? Can I do it with 5 lakh? No! You see if whatever I earn gets spent on rent and everyday expenses, what's the point of earning then? If [Doctor] Madam could fix the amount to at least 8 lakh, all of us could buy a house and save on the rent.

Puja, another veteran surrogate, advocated for a different procedure of "fixing" the amount—open negotiation between the surrogate and her client:

> Well to tell you the truth, this time I asked Madam to either get me a party that pays more or let me talk to my party myself. I've had two scissors [C-sections] now so this is my last opportunity. Madam got me this party and she says they will be paying me 4 lakh ($8,000). I wanted to ask for more but Madam and the client decided on the amount. If I could sit with them and talk, maybe they would have agreed to pay a lakh more. But Madam does not allow that.

While most veteran surrogates agree that open negotiation is desirable, currently such negotiations are explicitly discouraged by the doctors. But the demands for change were not limited to the economics of the surrogacy contract. Another recurring theme was their relationship with clients, especially the intended mother. In the earlier chapters of this study I explored the surrogates' belief that the couple hiring them would keep in touch even after delivery. In some cases the intended couple did, in fact, remain in touch. Anne continues to send her surrogate, Divya, e-mails, photographs, and gifts from California. The intended father from Spain is paying for the schooling of the children of his surrogate, Yashoda. Will sent a surprise gift to the husband of his surrogate, Salma—enough money for a motorcycle. Japanese client Jessy continues to "facebook" with her surrogate, Diksha, and occasionally sends pictures of their daughter, Muskaan. Diksha's post-delivery experience was unusually positive, partly because she had to take care of the baby for two months after delivery while the clients arranged for the necessary legal papers in Japan. Diksha beams as she tells me the story behind the baby's name, "Muskaan": "While she [the baby] was with us, we decided to name her 'Muskaan' [Hindi for "smile"]. That little girl made us smile! When they [the intended parents] came to pick her up they asked us what 'Muskaan' meant. When I explained the meaning to them, they started crying. A month later Jessy [intended mother] sent me an e-mail and told me that they have named the girl 'Emiko,' which means 'blessed and smiling child' in Japanese. She is an Indian Muskaan for me and a Japanese Muskaan for Jessy!"

In an earlier chapter I discussed how some symbolic gestures, for instance the intended mother calling the surrogate mother the baby's "mother," reflect the kin labor done by the women involved in surrogacy. In this case, respecting Diksha's choice of name for the baby is another form of kin labor performed by the intended mother. Diksha appreciates these gestures but is pragmatic about her relationship with Jessy—she recognizes that baby Muskaan may never really be aware that her other mother is in India.

But not all post-delivery stories are cordial. Many clients, apprehensive that the surrogate will change her mind about giving the baby away, prefer to sever all ties with the surrogate. These are the cases the surrogates label a "waste"—kin labor that has gone unrecognized and unreciprocated. Tejal was hired as a surrogate by a non-resident Indian couple settled in the United States. When I met Tejal in 2011, she recalled the delivery day rather bitterly:

> There was a lot of problem with the delivery and I had to have 15–20 bottles of IV in just two days. Ultimately I got a scissor [caesarean section]. I was unconscious when the couple came and took away the baby. They didn't even show it to my husband. The baby would have been three years today. But I don't even know what he looks like. I used to think they would invite us to America. I used to think of her as a sister—*all of it went to waste* [emphasis added]. Forget an invitation, they did not even call to see if we are dead or alive. They just finished their business, picked up the baby and left.

Although such experiences are not the norm, Tejal is not the only one to claim that her kin labor has been "wasted." Sudha delivered a baby for a couple from Mumbai, India. She recalls the day of the delivery:

> The couple and the family had become like a family to me. They treated me very well throughout the pregnancy. But on the day of the delivery their *tevar* [behavior] started changing. First they were reluctant to let me see the baby. When the nurses brought her over to me, she [the intended mother] started instructing the nurse to give me pills, to stop my breast milk! I had just delivered her baby and all she could think of is that I should not be allowed to feed the baby!

Surrogate Munni has a similar tale. Munni delivered a baby in 2007 for an Indian couple settled in the United States. Like Sudha, Munni is bewildered by the change in her client's behavior immediately after the delivery:

> My party was from America but they used to come to Garv often to visit their parents. They would call me every day from America and come visit me almost every month. They even allowed me to breast-feed the baby. They always said that when the baby grows up they would tell her about me—about her second mother in India. It's been over a year now; she would have been one year old last week. There have been no phone calls, nothing. I don't know what has gone wrong.

Munni seems surprised by the sudden severing of ties. Her relationship with her clients was unusually friendly while she was carrying their baby. But once she completed her contract, her reproduction became a classic example of alienated labor. Her clients honored the capitalist contract; they paid her and appropriated the surplus value of her reproductive labor—the baby.

The medical staff discourages the surrogates from making any attempts to remain in touch with their clients. For instance, an Indian surrogate told sociologist Arlie Hochschild (2012) that on the doctor's instructions, she deleted her client's phone number from her cell phone list. Teman (2010) reports similar instances in Israel, in which the hospital staff became "medical gatekeepers" in "institutionally" separating the surrogate from the newborn as well as from the intended mother (197). Despite these instructions, surrogates yearned for more contact. Most lamented that the "sisterly" ties that many surrogates established with the intended mother were terminated rather abruptly and the clients seldom stayed in touch. While all the six veteran surrogates agreed that clients often did not stay in touch, they were reluctant to comment on my second question: *Should* clients remain in touch with their surrogates?

Diksha hesitantly responds: "Well, I don't know. I don't know if I have the right to ask for anything. We [she points to the six "veteran" surrogates] have all fulfilled the contract. Of course I miss the baby and her [the client]. Of course I wish they would tell me more about her [the baby] and tell her about me. But I leave it to them. . . . Of course I would feel nice if they did."

Diksha is quick to clarify that "staying in touch" does not involve sending material gifts. The surrogates would expect only appreciation and respect: "We don't demand that they send us money. All we ask is that they treat us with respect. We bear babies for them. What we want in return is for them to talk to us nicely, treat us with respect. They should realize that because of us they have so much happiness in their house; they are being able to play with the baby, hold it, have it in their life. *I am talking about treating this woman with respect after the delivery, at least that much* [emphasis added]."

Diksha's response highlights a critical aspect of the surrogacy arrangement, one that is seldom discussed in mainstream debates—the dignity of surrogates. Apart from the material lack and want of food, livelihood, and housing, people living in poverty often describe their circumstances in terms of everyday indignities accentuated by their marginalization, voicelessness, and stigmatization.[10] For the surrogates at Garv, "change" implies not just an increase in the payments that they receive for their labor, but just as critically, an affirmation of their dignity as laborers. Diksha echoes the change demanded, albeit hesitantly, by some women— the desire that their kin labor does not go to waste and that clients continue to respect the ties they have forged across seemingly impossible borders of race, class, and nation.

Given the obvious gendered nature of this industry, an appealing aspiration is to envision solidarity among the women involved in surrogacy, whether they be the surrogates or the intended mothers. Over the years, the need to recognize diversity, situatedness, and multiplicity of experiences has been pushing feminists away from the concept of "global sisterhood" and toward the notion of "transnational feminisms." While the concept of global sisterhood allegedly glosses over the differences between women, "transnational feminisms" may have the potential to forge solidarity across the globe, among women of different positions and interests. In the seminal book *Feminism Without Borders: Decolonizing Theory, Practicing Solidarity* (2003a), Chandra Talpade Mohanty argues that for transnational feminisms to be possible, the politics of solidarity has to be based on "mutuality, accountability, and the recognition of common interests as the basis for relationships among diverse communities" (7). Sociologist Jyotsna Agnihotri Gupta (2006) applies this notion to new reproductive technologies to ask: "Can the need of infertile women for donor eggs or surrogacy services and the financial need of women that drives them to offer the same, thus creating a relationship of mutual dependency, be a basis for mutual solidarity?" (31). To make the leap from global sisterhood to transnational feminisms, the difficult task of envisioning a politics of solidarity cannot be left to the two sets of women involved in surrogacy—the surrogates and the intended mothers. Placing surrogacy and womb work within the continuum of reproductive labor, with sex work, care work, and other intimate forms of labor, may well be the first step toward imagining a broader community of women with common interests. A long overdue recognition of mutual dependencies, between sellers of reproductive labor and buyers of the same, is fundamental to an effective politics of solidarity.

EPILOGUE

DID THE "SPERM ON A RICKSHAW"
SAVE THE THIRD WORLD?

IN 2007, ten months after returning from the field, I had given up all hope of revisiting Garv and the Armaan Maternity Clinic. I had resigned myself to getting updates through e-mails and phone conversations with my informant friends. Then something happened that prompted me to plan another visit. One of the surrogacy hostels in India was featured in an episode of *The Oprah Winfrey Show*. The show portrayed the intended parents from the United States as nothing less than brave missionaries or cultural ambassadors,[1] while the surrogates were unambiguously portrayed as "women who had just won a lottery," a lottery that would change their lives. I watched the *Oprah* episode in Boston, and the simplistic portrayal of surrogacy irked me enough that I decided to rekindle my relationship with the doctor and the hostel matron. I returned to Garv in 2008 to revisit some of the women after their deliveries. I visited some in their village homes and others at their workplace. I met the repeat surrogates at the clinic and hostel. I returned to the field yet again in 2011.[2] Given the nationwide boom in the surrogacy industry, I was not surprised to find a flourishing fertility market in Garv. The clinic had grown in size. The doctor was expanding her operations and getting a multi-story hospital-hotel built that would house her international clients as well as the surrogates. The existing surrogacy hostels had expanded, and each hostel housed 70 pregnant women. To my surprise, I saw some familiar faces at both hostels. Some were women who were pregnant for the third time in five years, and others were former surrogates involved in the industry either as brokers or as nannies for international clients with newborn babies. The national and international media, the doctors, and the intended parents unanimously claim that surrogacy magically transforms the life of families living in desperate poverty. By revisiting the women I had previously interviewed, in this epilogue I ask a simple question: do the lives of surrogates, in fact, get transformed?

WHO COOKS THE DINNER?

The intended parents often gave cell phones to their surrogates who were living in surrogacy hostels. Late evenings at the hostel echoed with the voices of surrogates chatting with their children over the telephone: "Who cooked the dinner tonight?" Husbands' responses to their wives' peculiar work restrictions varied; some took over the household chores, at least temporarily, while others treated the nine months like a paid vacation. In my first year in the field, Divya's hostel was yet to be inaugurated, and surrogates resided in a makeshift dormitory above the clinic, staying there for only short periods of time—immediately after the embryo transfer and for a month before the delivery date. To prevent the surrogate from doing any household chores, Dr. Khanderia encouraged them to spend a substantial portion of their monthly allowances on paid domestic help at home. In some cases, the intended parents paid for such help. When domestic service was unaffordable, female kin—the surrogates' mother or mother-in-law—stepped in. Meena, a surrogate for clients from Mumbai, was planning to use the money to pay the mortgage for her husband's shop. When I met them in 2006, Meena's husband, Parag, accepted that he was not actively hunting for any job in the interim: "Well, she has been asked to just lie around and sleep. I decided to take a break as well. The money they [the intended parents] pay is not really enough for everything but we make do. . . . Now that she has been here [at the clinic] for the past three weeks, I have started doing some small things at home—like warming the milk for the children to drink and washing the dishes. My mother does the cooking and cleaning. I don't know all that."

In my second visit to the field, the living arrangement for surrogates had changed substantially. Most surrogates stayed in hostels for the entire length of their pregnancy, and the clients paid for their maintenance in the hostel. In most cases the husbands took responsibility for child care, while a neighbor or a female relative helped with housework. Rita, surrogate for the second time, says, "I have a very good husband. We decided not to tell my family that I am doing this the second time, so he does most of the housework. He takes care of the children, picks up and drops them to school, everything. In the beginning [of the pregnancy] when I was at home I did the cooking. I hired a maid for the cleaning, etc. I pay her with the monthly money they [the couple] pay us."

Razia, surrogate for clients from the United States, adds: "My husband takes care of the house nowadays. He manages everything—from cooking to child care. I taught him when I was at home right at the beginning of my pregnancy. He understands that I am suffering so much just to get some money for the family. I bear this pain and he bears the pain of household chores."

Do the men in the family continue to share the "pain of household chores" when the nine months of the contract are complete and the women go back home? In my second trip to the field I meet Razia again. She is at the clinic to meet her sister-in-law, another surrogate who is recovering from a caesarean delivery. Razia laughs when we start talking about her husband's household chores: "Well, what do you expect? It's back to normal. He started a small business with most of the money we earned. Two months ago he was unemployed and ready to take care of almost all the household chores. Now he is back to business. He does help me out with the children much more than before. He takes care of me much more as well!"

It seems to be "back to business" for other husbands as well. I meet surrogate Regina in the village a month after the delivery. Regina had a complicated delivery that left her very weak, but she is back to working as a part-time maid in people's houses. She complains about her husband, saying, "No, Amrita *didi*, not all husbands are bad. But my husband is an alcoholic and that's why I never give him the money I earn from cleaning houses. I have to run the house, feed the children, take all the responsibility. He knows nothing about housework. When I was in the clinic hostel, he started to help my son with the various chores. But now he just lies around. He knows I have saved some money and that makes him even more relaxed."

At the level of the household, men take on responsibility for household work only temporarily. While their wives stayed at the hostel, husbands learned some basic household chores and took some responsibility for child care. But there were others who treated their wives' surrogacy like a paid vacation and a possible passport to another country. When I met Salma in 2006, she was pregnant with twins for clients from New Jersey. Her husband, Faiz, used to be an auto-rickshaw driver, earning about Rs 2,500 ($50) per month. Faiz had left his job, and he spent most of his day sitting on the hostel porch or by his wife's bedside. He explained that he was taking a break from his driving and was preparing for a better job in the future: "I just got a passport made. I have been talking to Will [the intended father from New Jersey] about the possibility of working as a taxi driver somewhere in America. Will says a lot of Indians drive taxis there. If they call me to America I'll go and become a driver there. I can drive all kinds of cars and trucks."

Faiz was not alone in imagining that the intended parents would rescue him from poverty. In chapter 7 I discussed the inadvertent consequences of such aspirations—apart from being unrealistic, they inevitably reify notions of a rich (white) foreigner from the global north rescuing the hungry native from the Third World.

WHERE DID ALL THE MONEY GO?

Although the household division of labor does not get altered significantly, it seems reasonable to expect that the lump sum of money earned by the women will result in some long-term changes in the family. While most surrogates dream of building their own house and saving for their children's education and marriage, the actual outcome is often unpredictable.

Forty-five-year-old Savita, a cleaning lady at the clinic, was the first commercial surrogate at the clinic. Savita lived separately from her husband, with her daughter and son-in-law. In 2006, Dr. Khanderia persuaded Savita to become a surrogate for a client. Savita planned to quit the low-paying, backbreaking job at the clinic and use the money earned through surrogacy to live comfortably. She was confident that the money would change her life. A year after the delivery I bumped into her while she was sweeping the clinic courtyard. She revealed that there has been no improvement in her living standard and she continues to be a cleaning lady at the clinic: "I get paid such little money at this clinic that I had to use part of the money for daily purchases. I couldn't save anything. A lot of it went for my husband's treatment [medical expenses]. Then my granddaughter fell sick with tuberculosis and though I spent a lot in her treatment we couldn't save her. I did not ever want this, but now my daughter is also trying to become a surrogate."

The money earned through surrogacy could not get Savita and her family out of the cycle of poverty. Despite all her efforts, she was forced to allow her daughter to become a surrogate as well. Savita's story is not unusual. Many former surrogates reported that they spent their entire earnings on family medical expenses and their husbands' businesses. Nisha works as a nurse at the clinic and after persuading many women to become surrogates, she decided to try it herself: "I wanted to use the money to pay back the house loan and keep the rest to send my son to an English-medium school. But during my delivery my husband developed a kidney infection and then his business got mortgaged. After paying off the hospital bills and mortgage, I have almost nothing left for my son or our savings account."

Some surrogates, especially the women living with their in-laws, complained that their in-laws appropriated a major portion of the money, leaving almost nothing as savings. Anjali was a surrogate for clients from the United Kingdom. A year after her delivery, I visited her in her one-room hut in a village close to Garv.

> My husband doesn't have a fixed job and I am a housewife. We have no fixed income and were managing to survive with some money that my father-in-law got from his pension. I did this [surrogacy] basically for my two daughters, so that we could save for their education and marriage. But we stay here with my in-laws and they wanted to use the money to fix the house instead. I am illiterate and my husband is the one in control of the finances. I did not see even one rupee out of the one lakh [$2,000] I earned.

Sapna's story is identical to that of Anjali. But unlike Anjali, Sapna does not resent her in-laws for appropriating her money. Sapna was a surrogate for an Indian couple settled in the United States when I met her in 2006. Sapna's mother-in-law, Kanta (a surrogacy broker), had persuaded her to become a surrogate. I revisited Sapna two years later in their new house—her "contribution" to the family—and she told me:

> My father-in-law used the entire money to reconstruct this house and add another floor to it. I wanted to keep some money aside in a savings account but there is nothing left after the reconstruction. We [her husband and she] did not really want to use all the money on construction but my in-laws were very keen. My father-in-law managed all the surrogacy finances and he was the one taking the ultimate decision. It is fine. I feel good that I could help the family. Except for me, everyone else in this family works outside the house. This was my contribution.

Repeat surrogates and surrogates who were in abusive relationships or lived without their husbands were often less ambiguous about the benefits of the money earned. Dipali, a divorcée with two children, became a surrogate so that she could be self-sufficient. Dipali is also a self-proclaimed broker and recruits other women for egg donation to the clinic. On one such visit to the clinic Dipali talked about her financial situation a year after the delivery:

> I managed to build one room with the money I earned through surrogacy. I haven't yet moved out of my brother's house but I should be able to very soon. I am not spending any of the money for our daily expenses. I use the money I get as commission [she gets a commission of Rs 500 or $10 for each egg donor she brings to the clinic] to pay for my children's everyday expenses. My brother still pays for their school but once I become a surrogate again, I will be able to take care of them.

The only other single parent was surrogate Yashoda, a widow living with her abusive in-laws. Although I was unable to get in touch with Yashoda after she delivered twins to a single man from Spain, her broker, Vimla, informed me that Yashoda managed to move out of her in-laws' house to a rented hut in another village.

Rita, a repeat surrogate, talked confidently about the benefits of her earnings:

> I have a very good husband. He consults me before any decision. But I have a sister-in-law who is a real *khoonchoos* [stingy person]. The first time [that Rita became a surrogate] she was taking care of my children but she wanted to know how each and every paisa [fraction of the rupee] was spent. She lives in another village so the second time I told him [her husband] not to tell her. We have saved the money from my second surrogacy. I am using the savings for my daughter's education and partly for reconstruction.

Puja, is another repeat surrogate, and by 2011 she had delivered babies for an Indian couple, a Canadian woman, and was undergoing treatment to become a surrogate for a couple from South India. In my first meeting with her, in 2006, Puja had spoken enthusiastically about her dreams: "I always wanted to have a house of my own, a house with running water, you know . . . don't laugh, I wanted to become an air hostess. I want to go abroad, to America. . . . My family always jokes about my plans. . . . They keep saying that *main hawa mein baatein karti hun* [I am talking in the air]. They think I am too ambitious. But I will show them."

I met Puja at the clinic the following year, when she was undergoing treatment to become a surrogate for the second time. She had managed to build herself a house with the money she had earned from her first surrogacy contract. Although she had abandoned her plans of "going abroad," she was confident that her second surrogacy would pay enough for another plot of land that she could give as dowry at her daughter's wedding. Four years later, I run into Puja once again, this time at the new hostel. Although she greets me with her usual "high five" and grin, I can see that she is not as fiery anymore. She has dark circles under her eyes and admits that she feels exhausted.

> You must be laughing and thinking, "Every time I come here, this Puja is pregnant again!" But what should I do? This inflation does not allow me to stop [becoming a surrogate]. Earlier you could get a milk carton for Rs 5 [10 cents]. Now it's double that amount. When guests come to your house, you have to think twice before you serve them even tea. My children's school fees double every year. I already spend so much on their fees, their uniform, and their books. When my daughter finishes her high school she wants to join a medical school. I will have to use the money I get this time from surrogacy to pay "donation" to her college. No college gives admission for free nowadays; you have to bribe your way in.

When I ask Puja about her dream of becoming an air hostess, and of traveling to foreign lands, she laughs: "Yes, I wanted to become an air hostess. I don't know why. I guess I had the fire in me to do something grand. As you can see, I could not do anything grand. I am pinning all my hopes on my daughter now. I hope God lets her achieve something grand. I pray that my daughter can really become a doctor one day, move to America and work and live there. I pray every day that she does not have to do for her daughter what I had to do for her."

Much like other surrogates, Puja has abandoned her own "grand" dreams of going abroad and saving up for a comfortable future. But she holds on to her dream that the money she earns from her last surrogacy will allow her daughter to live a more comfortable life.

While my first trip had challenged many of my own preconceived notions about surrogacy, most of my assumptions about the long-term effects of surrogacy remained unchallenged by my next two visits. As I had predicted, surrogacy was not much of a "lottery"—the lives of most surrogates did not change. Some were able to have more control over their earnings than others, but few were able to save up enough to get out of the cycle of poverty. In most cases, the money was used up for health emergencies, one-time constructions, and family businesses, and had little effect on everyday life.

In the determined pursuit of a (feminist) fairy-tale ending, I close this section with one of the most exhilarating and unexpected stories. Surrogacy did transform the lives of at least two women—Mansi and Mona. Mansi's dream was to start a beauty parlor with her colleague and roommate at the hostel, Mona. In my last visit to the field, a nurse informed me that both of them were working as trainees in a small parlor in Garv. Both women were able to use the networks formed in the hostel as well as the "training" received to get involved in further employment outside the house. I invite Mansi to the café that sells her favorite snack. She enthusiastically relates her future plans:

> The money [from surrogacy] is not as much, you know. It seems like it would be enough for 10 years but it actually is nothing. Life is very expensive nowadays. But Mona and I both have managed to keep some money aside for this [their parlor]. I hope it is enough. We want something small, maybe start with just two of us, and then hire more women? Manicure, *mehendi* [henna], and putting flowers in women's hair. . . . There is demand for parlors here everywhere, you know. If we can keep this going, we can even one day do bridal makeups. Mona and I have learnt some of these things already. Amrita *didi*, can you suggest a name for our parlor?

APPENDIX A

SELECTED CLAUSES FROM THE ASSISTED REPRODUCTIVE TECHNOLOGIES (REGULATION) DRAFT BILL, 2010

CLAUSE 34. RIGHTS AND DUTIES IN RELATION TO SURROGACY

(1) Both the couple or individual seeking surrogacy through the use of assisted reproductive technology, and the surrogate mother, shall enter into a surrogacy agreement which shall be legally enforceable.

(2) All expenses, including those related to insurance if available, of the surrogate related to a pregnancy achieved in furtherance of assisted reproductive technology shall, during the period of pregnancy and after delivery as per medical advice, and till the child is ready to be delivered as per medical advice, to the biological parent or parents, shall be borne by the couple or individual seeking surrogacy.

(3) Notwithstanding anything contained in sub-section (2) of this section and subject to the surrogacy agreement, the surrogate mother may also receive monetary compensation from the couple or individual, as the case may be, for agreeing to act as such surrogate.

(4) A surrogate mother shall relinquish all parental rights over the child.

(5) No woman less than twenty one years of age and over thirty five years of age shall be eligible to act as a surrogate mother under this Act. Provided that no woman shall act as a surrogate for more than five successful live births in her life, including her own children.

(6) Any woman seeking or agreeing to act as a surrogate mother shall be medically tested for such diseases, sexually transmitted or otherwise, as may be prescribed, and all other communicable diseases which may

endanger the health of the child, and must declare in writing that she has not received a blood transfusion or a blood product in the last six months.

(7) Individuals or couples may obtain the service of a surrogate through an ART bank, which may advertise to seek surrogacy provided that no such advertisement shall contain any details relating to the caste, ethnic identity or descent of any of the parties involved in such surrogacy. No assisted reproductive technology clinic shall advertise to seek surrogacy for its clients.

(8) A surrogate mother shall, in respect of all medical treatments or procedures in relation to the concerned child, register at the hospital or such medical facility in her own name, clearly declare herself to be a surrogate mother, and provide the name or names and addresses of the person or persons, as the case may be, for whom she is acting as a surrogate, along with a copy of the certificate mentioned in clause 17 below.

(9) If the first embryo transfer has failed in a surrogate mother, she may, if she wishes, decide to accept on mutually agreed financial terms, at most two more successful embryo transfers for the same couple that had engaged her services in the first instance. No surrogate mother shall undergo embryo transfer more than three times for the same couple.

(10) The birth certificate issued in respect of a baby born through surrogacy shall bear the name(s) of individual/individuals who commissioned the surrogacy, as parents.

(11) The person or persons who have availed of the services of a surrogate mother shall be legally bound to accept the custody of the child/children irrespective of any abnormality that the child/children may have, and the refusal to do so shall constitute an offence under this Act.

(12) Subject to the provisions of this Act, all information about the surrogate shall be kept confidential and information about the surrogacy shall not be disclosed to anyone other than the central database of the Department of Health Research, except by an order of a court of competent jurisdiction.

(13) A surrogate mother shall not act as an oocyte donor for the couple or individual, as the case may be, seeking surrogacy.

(14) No assisted reproductive technology clinic shall provide information on or about surrogate mothers or potential surrogate mothers to any person.

(15) Any assisted reproductive technology clinic acting in contravention of sub-section 14 of this section shall be deemed to have committed an offence under this Act.

(16) In the event that the woman intending to be a surrogate is married, the consent of her spouse shall be required before she may act as such surrogate.

(17) A surrogate mother shall be given a certificate by the person or persons who have availed of her services, stating unambiguously that she has acted as a surrogate for them.

(18) A relative, a known person, as well as a person unknown to the couple may act as a surrogate mother for the couple/individual. In the case of a relative acting as a surrogate, the relative should belong to the same generation as the women desiring the surrogate.

(19) A foreigner or foreign couple not resident in India, or a non-resident Indian individual or couple, seeking surrogacy in India shall appoint a local guardian who will be legally responsible for taking care of the surrogate during and after the pregnancy as per clause 34.2, till the child/children are delivered to the foreigner or foreign couple or the local guardian. Further, the party seeking the surrogacy must ensure and establish to the assisted reproductive technology clinic through proper documentation (a letter from either the embassy of the Country in India or from the foreign ministry of the Country, clearly and unambiguously stating that (a) the country permits surrogacy, and (b) the child born through surrogacy in India, will be permitted entry in the Country as a biological child of the commissioning couple/individual) that the party would be able to take the child/children born through surrogacy, including where the embryo was a consequence of donation of an oocyte or sperm, outside of India to the country of the party's origin or residence as the case may be. If the foreign party seeking surrogacy fails to take delivery of the child born to the surrogate mother commissioned by the foreign party, the local guardian shall be legally obliged to take delivery of the child and be free to hand the child over to an adoption agency, if the commissioned party or their legal representative fails to claim the child within one months of the birth of the child. During the transition period, the local guardian shall be responsible for the well-being of the child. In case of adoption or the legal guardian having to bring up the child, the child will be given Indian citizenship.

(20) A couple or an individual shall not have the service of more than one surrogate at any given time.

(21) A couple shall not have simultaneous transfer of embryos in the woman and in a surrogate.

(22) Only Indian citizens shall have a right to act as a surrogate, and no ART bank/ART clinics shall receive or send an Indian for surrogacy abroad.

(23) Any woman agreeing to act as a surrogate shall be duty-bound not to engage in any act that would harm the foetus during pregnancy and the child after birth, until the time the child is handed over to the designated person(s).

(24) The commissioning parent(s) shall ensure that the surrogate mother and the child she deliver are appropriately insured until the time the child is handed over to the commissioning parent(s) or any other person as per the agreement and till the surrogate mother is free of all health complications arising out of surrogacy.

CLAUSE 35. DETERMINATION OF STATUS OF THE CHILD

(1) A child born to a married couple through the use of assisted reproductive technology shall be presumed to be the legitimate child of the couple, having been born in wedlock and with the consent of both spouses, and shall have identical legal rights as a legitimate child born through sexual intercourse.

(2) A child born to an unmarried couple through the use of assisted reproductive technology, with the consent of both the parties, shall be the legitimate child of both parties.

(3) In the case of a single woman the child will be the legitimate child of the woman, and in the case of a single man the child will be the legitimate child of the man.

(4) In case a married or unmarried couple separates or gets divorced, as the case may be, after both parties consented to the assisted reproductive technology treatment but before the child is born, the child shall be the legitimate child of the couple.

(5) A child born to a woman artificially inseminated with the stored sperm of her dead husband shall be considered as the legitimate child of the couple.

(6) If a donated ovum contains ooplasm from another donor ovum, both the donors shall be medically tested for such diseases, sexually transmitted or otherwise, as may be prescribed, and all other communicable diseases which may endanger the health of the child, and the donor of both

the ooplasm and the ovum shall relinquish all parental rights in relation to such child.

(7) The birth certificate of a child born through the use of assisted reproductive technology shall contain the name or names of the parent or parents, as the case may be, who sought such use.

(8) If a foreigner or a foreign couple seeks sperm or egg donation, or surrogacy, in India, and a child is born as a consequence, the child, even though born in India, shall not be an Indian citizen.

CLAUSE 36. RIGHT OF THE CHILD TO INFORMATION ABOUT DONORS OR SURROGATES

(1) A child may, upon reaching the age of 18, ask for any information, excluding personal identification, relating to the donor or surrogate mother.

(2) The legal guardian of a minor child may apply for any information, excluding personal identification, about his/her genetic parent or parents or surrogate mother when required, and to the extent necessary, for the welfare of the child.

(3) Personal identification of the genetic parent or parents or surrogate mother may be released only in cases of life threatening medical conditions which require physical testing or samples of the genetic parent or parents or surrogate mother. Provided that such personal identification will not be released without the prior informed consent of the genetic parent or parents or surrogate mother.

APPENDIX B

CONSENT FORM TO BE SIGNED BY SURROGATES

Surrogates at the Armaan Maternity Clinic and their husbands sign or put a thumbprint on the consent form below. This form is the one suggested by the Indian Council of Medical Research (available for download at http://icmr.nic.in/art/Chapter_4.pdf).

4.7 AGREEMENT FOR SURROGACY

I, _____ (the woman), with the consent of my husband (name), of _____ (address) have agreed to act as a host mother for the couple, _____ _____ (wife) and_____ (husband), both of whom are unable (or do not wish to) to have a child by any other means. I had a full discussion with _____of the clinic on _____ in regard to the matter of my acting as a surrogate mother for the child of the above couple.

I understand that the methods of treatment may include:

1. Stimulation of the genetic mother for follicular recruitment

2. The recovery of one or more oocytes from the genetic mother by ultrasound-guided oocyte recovery or by laparoscopy.

3. The fertilisation of the oocytes from the genetic mother with the sperm of her husband or an anonymous donor.

4. The fertilisation of a donor oocyte by the sperm of the husband.

5. The maintenance and storage by cryopreservation of the embryo resulting from such fertilisation until, in the view of the medical and scientific staff, it is ready for transfer.

6. Implantation of the embryo obtained through any of the above possibilities into my uterus, after the necessary treatment if any.

I have been assured that the genetic mother and the genetic father have been screened for HIV and hepatitis B and C before oocyte recovery and found to be seronegative for all these diseases. I have, however, been also informed that there is a small risk of the mother or/and the father becoming seropositive for HIV during the window period.

I consent to the above procedures and to the administration of such drugs that may be necessary to assist in preparing my uterus for embryos transfer, and for support in the luteal phase.

I understand and accept that there is no certainty that a pregnancy will result from these procedures.

I understand and accept that the medical and scientific staff can give no assurance that any pregnancy will result in the delivery of a normal and living child.

I am unrelated/related (relation) _____ to the couple (the would-be genetic parents).

I have worked out the financial terms and conditions of the surrogacy with the couple in writing and an appropriately authenticated copy of the agreement has been filed with the clinic, which the clinic will keep confidential.

I agree to hand over the child to _____ and _____ , the couple (to _____ in case of their separation during my pregnancy, or to the survivor in case of the death of one of them during pregnancy) as soon as I am permitted to do so by the Hospital/Clinic/Nursing home where the child is delivered.

I undertake to inform the ART clinic, _____, of the result of the pregnancy.

I take no responsibility that the child delivered by me will be normal in all respects. I understand that the biological parents of the child have a legal obligation to accept their child that I deliver and that the child would have all the inheritance rights of a child of the biological parents as per the prevailing law.

I will not be asked to go through sex determination tests for the child during the pregnancy and that I have the full right to refuse such tests.

I understand that I would have the right to terminate the pregnancy at my will; I will then refund all certified and documented expenses incurred on the pregnancy by the biological parents or their representative. If, however, the pregnancy has to be terminated on expert medical advice, these expenses will not be refunded.

I have been tested for HIV, hepatitis B and C and shown to be seronegative for these viruses just before embryo transfer.

I certify that (a) I have not had any drug intravenously administered into me through a shared syringe; (b) I have not undergone blood transfusion; and (c) I and my husband have had no extramarital relationship in the last six months.

I also declare that I will not use drugs intravenously, undergo blood transfusion excepting of blood obtained through a certified blood bank, and avoid sexual intercourse during the pregnancy.

I undertake not to disclose the identity of the couple.

In the case of the death of both the husband and wife (the couple) during my pregnancy, I will deliver the child to _____ or _____ in this order; I will be provided, before the embryo transfer into me, a written agreement of the above persons to accept the child in the case of the above-mentioned eventuality.

ENDORSEMENT BY THE ART CLINIC

I/we have personally explained to _____ and _____ the details and implications of his/her/their signing this consent/approval form, and made sure to the extent humanly possible that he/she/they understand these details and implications.

Signed:

(Surrogate Mother)

Name, Address and Signature of the Witness from the clinic

Name and Signature of the Doctor

APPENDIX C: DESCRIPTIVE TABLES

TABLE AP.1 Surrogates at Armaan Clinic

NAME	AGE	RELIGION	WORK	HUSBAND'S WORK	INCOME PER MONTH ($)	EDUCATION	CHILDREN	COMMISSIONING PARENT(S) FROM
SUDHA	27	Hindu	Farmer	Truck driver	30	Primary school	1	India
DIVYA	30	Hindu	Bank teller	Bank teller	200	College	2	United States
MEENA	26	Hindu	Housewife	Hair salon	60	Middle school	3	India
PUJA	27	Hindu	Works in a store	Painter	50	High school	2	United States
SALMA	25	Muslim	Housewife	Driver	50	Middle school	2	United States
DIPALI	25	Hindu	Insurance agent	Divorced	30	High school	2	South Africa
VANEETA	36	Christian	Staff nurse	Tailor	150	Primary school	3	United States
VIDYA	30	Christian	Housewife	Daily laborer	40	High school	3	India
DAKSHA	20	Hindu	Housewife	Farmer	20	Illiterate	3	India
ANJALI	25	Christian	Housewife	No fixed job	20	Primary school	2	United Kingdom
PARVATI	36	Hindu	Nurse	Factory worker	100	Primary school	1	India
GAURI	28	Hindu	Housewife	Salesman	30	Illiterate	2	United States

TABLE AP.1 (continued)

NAME	AGE	RELIGION	WORK	HUSBAND'S WORK	INCOME PER MONTH ($)	EDUCATION	CHILDREN	COMMISSIONING PARENT(S) FROM
JAGRUTI	35	Hindu	Works in a school	Haircutter	35	Middle school	3	India
KRITI	23	Hindu	Housewife	Vendor	40	Middle school	2	United States
TEJAL	27	Hindu	Housewife	Painter	30	Middle school	2	United States
SAPNA	27	Hindu	Housewife	Factory worker	120	Primary school	2	United States
SAVITA	45	Hindu	Cleans the clinic	Separated	40	Primary school	2	Singapore
HETAL	35	Hindu	Floor supervisor	Contractor	150	High school	2	India
JYOTI	26	Hindu	Housewife and tailor	Auto-rickshaw driver	50	High school	3	United States
REGINA	45	Christian	Maid	Rickshaw puller	30	Illiterate	2	United States
VARSHA	38	Hindu	Waitress	Unemployed	15	Middle school	2	India
RITA	29	Hindu	Housewife	Plastic collector	60	Primary school	2	United States
MUNNI	35	Hindu	Nanny	Unemployed	40	Middle school	3	United States
NISHA	36	Christian	Nurse	Auto driver	100	Middle school	1	United States
YASHODA	38	Christian	Clinic maid	Deceased	20	Illiterate	2	Spain

Name	Age	Religion				Education		Location
SEJAL	30	Hindu	Teacher	Painter	40	High school	1	Dubai
TINA	26	Christian	Housewife	Auto driver	60	Middle school	3	Dubai
RINA	26	Hindu	Works in store	Auto driver	100	High school	2	United States
MANSI	29	Hindu	Tailor	Tailor	50	High school	2	Sri Lanka
MONA	24	Hindu	Housewife	Factory worker	70	High school	2	United States
VAISHALI	24	Hindu	Cook	Factory worker	70	High school	1	United States
SHANTA	33	Hindu	Works in a parlor	Auto driver	100	Middle school	3	United States
NASEEM	30	Muslim	Housewife	Daily laborer	40	Middle school	1	India
PANNA	27	Hindu	Housewife	Vendor	60	Middle school	3	Turkey
NAINA	36	Christian	Nurse	Factory worker	60	High school	2	United States
SHARDA	38	Christian	Housewife	Mill worker	40	Middle school	3	India
GEETA	35	Hindu	Housewife	Farmer	200	Illiterate	2	Does not know
RAZIA	25	Muslim	Sorts out plastic	Unemployed	15	Middle school	2	United States
RAMYA	29	Hindu	Bank teller	Factory worker	70	High school	1	United States
SANGEETA	33	Hindu	Housewife	Watchman	30	Illiterate	2	India
HASOMATI	30	Hindu	Housewife	Mill worker	40	Middle school	2	Dubai
DIKSHA	24	Hindu	Nanny	Factory worker	70	Middle school	2	Japan

TABLE AP.2 Contraceptive Use and Caesarean Sections at Armaan, 2007

NAME	AGE	CHILDREN	CONTRACEPTIVE USE	DELIVERY OF OWN CHILD(REN)	DELIVERY OF SURROGATE BABY
SUDHA	27	1	None (rhythm method)	Vaginal, in hospital	C-section
DIVYA	30	2	Yes (IUD)	1 Vaginal, 1 C-section	C-section
MEENA	26	3	No (rhythm method)	Vaginal, midwife at home	C-section
PUJA	27	2	Yes (sterilization)	Vaginal	2 C-sections
SALMA	25	2	Yes (IUD)	Vaginal, midwife at home	C-section
DIPALI	25	2	Yes (sterilization)	Vaginal	C-section
VANEETA	36	3	Yes (sterilization)	Vaginal, midwife at home	C-section
VIDYA	30	3	No (rhythm method)	Vaginal, midwife at home	C-section
DAKSHA	20	3	No	Vaginal, midwife at home	vaginal
ANJALI	25	2	No	Vaginal, midwife at home	C-section
PARVATI	36	1	No	Vaginal, in hospital	C-section
GAURI	28	2	Yes (sterilization)	Vaginal, midwife at home	C-section
JAGRUTI	35	3	No (rhythm method)	Vaginal, in hospital	C-section
TEJAL	30	1	Yes (IUD)	C-section	C-section
SAPNA	27	2	No	Vaginal, in hospital	C-section
SAVITA	45	2	Yes (sterilization)	Vaginal, midwife at home	C-section

NAME	AGE	CHILDREN	CONTRACEPTIVE USE	DELIVERY OF OWN CHILD(REN)	DELIVERY OF SURROGATE BABY
HETAL	35	2	No (rhythm method)	Vaginal, in hospital	C-section
JYOTI	26	3	Yes (pills)	Vaginal, midwife at home	C-section
REGINA	42	2	Yes (sterilization)	Vaginal, at home with kin assistance	C-section
VARSHA	38	2	No (rhythm method)	Vaginal, midwife at home	C-section
RITA	29	2	Yes (pills)	Vaginal, in hospital	vaginal
MUNNI	35	3	No	Vaginal, midwife at home	C-section
NISHA	36	1	Yes (sterilization)	Vaginal, in hospital	C-section
YASHODA	38	2	——	Vaginal, at home with kin assistance	C-section
TINA	26	3	Yes	Vaginal, midwife at home	C-section
RINA	26	2	Yes	Vaginal, in hospital	Yet to deliver (2007)
MANSI	29	2	No	Vaginal, nurse at home	C-section
MONA	24	2	No	Vaginal, in hospital	C-section
VAISHALI	24	1	No	C-section	C-section
SHANTA	33	3	Yes (sterilization)	Vaginal, at parents' home	C-section
NASEEM	30	1	Yes (sterilization)	Vaginal, at home with kin assistance	C-section

NAME	AGE	CHILDREN	CONTRACEPTIVE USE	DELIVERY OF OWN CHILD(REN)	DELIVERY OF SURROGATE BABY
PANNA	27	3	No	Vaginal, at home with kin assistance	C-section
NAINA	36	2	Yes (sterilization)	Vaginal, at home with kin assistance	C-section
SHARDA	38	4	Yes (sterilization)	Vaginal, at home with kin assistance	C-section
GEETA	35	2	No	Vaginal, midwife at home	C-section
RAZIA	25	2	No	Vaginal, at home with kin assistance	C-section
RAMYA	29	1	Yes (sterilization)	Vaginal, in hospital	C-section
SANGEETA	33	2	Yes (sterilization)	Vaginal, at home with kin assistance	C-section
HASOMATI	30	2	No (rhythm method)	Vaginal, at home with kin assistance	— Yet to deliver (2007)
DIKSHA	24	2	No	Vaginal	C-section

NOTES

1. INTRODUCTION: WOMBS IN LABOR

1. This chilling depiction of surrogacy in Atwood's fictional Republic of Gilead provides a vision of what many feminists in the late twentieth century believed would soon be reality if the new reproductive technologies proceeded unchecked. Children would be thought of exclusively as products. A class of women would be valuable merely as breeders. Atwood describes the gymnasium-turned-dormitory where the handmaids-in-training slept on old military cots and were watched continuously by Aunts with cattle prods.

2. I have chosen a fictitious name for the city primarily to protect the identities of my subjects. I refrain from using the real name also because I do not want this book to serve as "publicity," in any form, for the doctor or the clinic.

3. In her incisive work on new reproductive technologies, Charis Thompson (2005, 57) describes two phases of feminist engagement with new reproductive technologies (NRT) like surrogacy: Phase 1 encompasses 1980–1991 and Phase 2 covers 1992–2000. According to Thompson, Phase 1 is characterized by influential feminist writings on the "excessive medicalization of reproduction in the global north and the crisis it posed for women." The landmark research during this phase included works by Emily Martin (2001) and Barbara Katz Rothman (1982, 1986, and 1989). This phase saw a call for the rejection of these patriarchal technologies and "a reclaiming of natural childbirth by and for women." The global dimensions of some of these writings can be seen in the critique of prenatal testing and female feticide in India, concerns about sterilization, testing, and dumping of dubious drugs on consumers in the global south. For instance, a resolution passed by FINRAGE (Feminist International Network of Resistance to Reproductive and Genetic Engineering) in the 1980s called for "a different kind of science that respected the dignity of womankind." The predominant message at this time, echoed by FINRAGE, was that it was "not too late to say 'no' to these technologies (Thompson 2005, 59). The second phase witnesses a gradual shift away from the "moral certainty" of the writings in the 1980s to "a tone of moral ambivalence" about NRTs. Instead of the monolithic opposition to

NRTs, there was now a focus on the lived world of users of NRTs, the multiplicities of women's experiences, and the potential of NRTs to disrupt conventional gender and familial roles. Much like the scholarship on other NRTs, over time there has been some dilution of the moral certainty about the need to reject surrogacy practices. But anxiety about the practice continues to dominate the literature even today.

4. For a less dystopian depiction of surrogacy see the predictions made about the use of black women's wombs within gestational surrogacy by Dorothy Roberts (2009). Also see Sandra Harding's predictions that "the Baby M case could be the forerunner of the use of poor and third world women's wombs to produce children for economically advantaged European American couples" (1991, 203).

5. Some recent discussions on the surrogacy industry in India include two chapters in Arlie Hochschild's (2012) book *The Outsourced Self: Intimate Life in Market Times*, based on interviews with one set of intended parents and surrogates in two Indian clinics. Other works based on narratives of surrogates include Kalindi Vora's article in *Scholar and Feminist Online* (Vora 2010), Sharmila Rudrappa's ongoing work with surrogate mothers in Bangalore (2012), Sayantani DasGupta and Shamita Das Dasgupta's edited book on gestational surrogate mothers in India (2014), and Rebecca Haimowitz and Vaishali Sinha's documentary *Made in India* (2010), which follows the journey of a white, middle-class couple from the United States to a fertility clinic in India and includes some conversations with their surrogate. There are other works, for instance by women's health and reproductive rights activists like the Delhi-based organization SAMA and writings by activist Imrana Qadeer, which are as important. I conduct a comparative analysis with relevant findings of these studies in the empirical chapters of this book.

6. Reproductive labor is typically defined as activities such as purchasing household goods, preparing and serving food, laundering and repairing clothing, socializing children, providing care and emotional support (Glenn 1992). While surrogate motherhood does not fall under the usual definition of reproductive labor, I have previously argued that with globalization and ever-expanding reproductive technology, "gestational services" need to be added to the list of care work (Pande 2010b). In their edited book *Intimate Labors: Cultures, Technologies, and the Politics of Care* (2010), Eileen Boris and Rhacel Salazar Parreñas build on feminist scholarship on reproductive labor to examine "the social construction of commodified intimacies" (7). The umbrella term "intimate labor" brings under its ambit a continuum of gendered forms of labor that involve "embodied and affective interactions in the service of social reproduction." For instance, Laura Briggs, writing about international adoption markets in the same volume, argues that meeting one's intimate needs would include not only child care but also the bearing of children for others, what she calls "offshore reproduction."

7. See Satz (1992) for more on the thesis that there ought to be an asymmetry between our treatment of reproductive labor and our treatment of other forms of labor.

8. According to Nancy Fraser (2011), such a "defensive project" takes attention away from the historical fact that long before these were "marketised," social construction of such labor as non-commodities was typically a source of domination.

9. Here, I am particularly mindful of Alison Bailey's caution against a "single-pointed focus on 'choice.'" Such a focus, Bailey believes, "occidentalizes Indian surrogacy work . . . and obscures the injustices behind these choices" (2011, 9). Instead of "obscuring" injustices, this book provides a systematic evaluation of the choices made by the surrogates so as to reveal the true nature and complexity of these layers of power.

10. See Hollander and Einwohner (2004) for a useful seven-part typology of resistance.

11. In the absence of a national registry, there is no reliable information on the number of ART clinics offering surrogacy in India. Some recent studies have estimated the industry to be worth as much as $400 million (Kohli 2011). Many Indian clinics report that surrogacy arrangements have doubled in the past decade, with most of the demand coming from international clients and non-resident Indians. According to the National Commission for Women, there are about 3,000 clinics across India currently offering surrogacy services (Kannan 2009). But there are 30,000 infertility clinics in total (Krishnakumar 2003), which means that it is reasonable to predict that 27,000 more have the potential to launch surrogacy practices. Moreover, there are countless other clinics currently offering surrogacy services without registering with any regulatory authority. See Shuriah Niazi, "Surrogacy Boom," BOLOJI, October 14, 2007, http://www.boloji.com/wfs6/wfs1027.htm; "Wombs for Rent in a Hamlet of Hope," *Asian Pacific Post*, March 9, 2006, http://www.asianpacificpost.com/portal2/ffB0808109dc23b20109dc491ba8001a_Wombs-for rent in a hamlet of hope.do.html; Amelia Gentleman, "India Nurtures Business of Surrogate Motherhood," *New York Times*, March 10, 2008, http://www.nytimes.com/2008/03/ 10/world/asia/ 10surrogate.html.

12. In the United States, clients of commercial surrogacy can expect to pay a total amount between $60,000 and $100,000. The gestational surrogate gets between $20,000 and $25,000, donor eggs cost $4,500 on average, and donor sperm typically cost $300 on average (Twine 2011). In India, the breakdown is estimated to be $2,500 to $7,000 as surrogacy fees, $100 to $150 for donor eggs, and total costs reportedly between $20,000 and $35,000.

13. See Markens (2007, 24) for a tabular summary of comparative international laws on surrogacy.

14. The majority of medical travelers to India are cardiac patients, but an increasing number of patients are coming for joint replacement, plastic surgery, and eye treatment. Reproductive travel—including all treatments that involve medical and scientific manipulation of human gametes and embryos in order to produce a term pregnancy—is the latest addition to this ever-growing list of services. The usual reasons for reproductive travel are that the treatment is forbidden in the home country for moral/religious reasons; treatment is not available because of lack of expertise or equipment; treatment is not available because it is not considered safe enough; certain categories of patients are not eligible for assisted reproduction; the waiting lists are too long in the home country; and the costs to be paid by the patients are too high in the home country.

15. A 2013 news report indicates that the "anti-gay" clause added that year by India's Ministry of Home Affairs has prompted many international gay clients from countries like Australia and Israel to seek alternative destinations like Thailand for commercial surrogates. http://www.abc.net.au/news/2013–04–13/thai-surrogacy-concerns/4624388.

16. For a detailed analysis of U.S.-India citizenship laws regarding ARTS and surrogacy, see Smerdon 2008–2009.

17. For more details about the artistic work done by Global Stories, see www.globalstories.net.

18. In her ongoing work on surrogates in Bangalore, India Sharmila Rudrappa reports that while most of her interviewees were "in debt," they were not among the poorest. In fact, most were factory workers earning "more than the average woman in the city" (2012, 22). In her study of surrogacy in two Indian clinics, Sheela Saravanan reports that most of her 13 respondents were "on the edge of poverty either because they were in debt or homeless" (2010, 27). More study on the surrogacy services mushrooming in many different cities in India is required to determine the (possibly changing) demography of commercial surrogates.

2. PRO-NATAL TECHNOLOGIES IN AN ANTI-NATAL STATE

1. Lock and Kaufert (2000) compare and contrast the responses of women in many countries in the global south to modern medical technologies.

2. A 2010 Save the Children report ranks India first in the number of maternal deaths, with more than 68,000 women dying each year from complications during or after childbirth. These deaths are reported to be partly due to lack of qualified care. Only 13 percent of low-income women give birth in any kind of formal health facility, and trained professionals assist at only one in seven home births. http://www.savethechildren.org/atf/cf/%7B9def2ebe-10ae-432c-9bd0-df91d2eba74a%7D/SOWM-2010-Women-on-the-Front-Lines-of-Health-Care.pdf.

3. In addition to the urban/rural dimension, there are regional dimensions to the history of biomedicalization in India. Some states in Southern India have better human and gender development indices than the national average. These states experience comparatively low maternal deaths and a relatively higher use of maternal care services. For instance, Cecilia van Hollen's work in Chennai, Tamil Nadu, suggests that in the 1990s women from lower economic classes and urban slum dwellers used available obstetric and prophylactic technology extensively. Hollen indicates that the use of these invasive medical technologies were as much a reflection of the women's agency as their governability.

4. The national emergency was a 19-month period between 1975 and 1977 when the president of India, upon the advice of Prime Minister Indira Gandhi, declared a state of emergency. Effectively this allowed Gandhi to suspend elections and all civil liberties.

5. Depo-Provera, an injectable hormonal contraceptive manufactured by a U.S. pharmaceutical firm, has often been at the center of contraceptive controversy. According to health activist and social scientist Betsy Hartmann, the primary "advantage" of this contraceptive is the way it is administered—a single shot needs to be given to a woman every three to six months. Hartmann (1995, 199) writes: "For women in India, whose husbands object to their using birth control, Depo can be given surreptitiously, during a quick visit to or by a family planning worker." But as Hartmann points out, unlike the pill or condom, a long-term contraceptive like Depo means complete "loss of control—even if a woman suffers some adverse effects from Depo (which can range from headaches, nausea to a possible link to breast, endometrial, and cervical cancers), there is nothing she can do until the injection wears off." In addition, Depo can be associated with the "injection mystique"—people in India associating injections with "safe, effective, modern medicine, which they are eager to receive." This trust in modern medicine, especially injections, makes it easier to administer Depo without explaining its side effects (Hartmann 1995, 199).

6. For a systematic analysis of the transitions in the Indian state's healthcare priorities and policies since the 1950s, see Qadeer 2010b.

7. Roberts recognizes that policy regulations add a class dimension to this racial disparity. For instance, Medicaid does not promote in vitro fertilization for poor infertile couples, irrespective of their race.

8. The few existing studies on infertility in India indicate that the incidence of total infertility in the country is around 8 to 10 percent, and for the vast majority of Indian women it is preventable, as it is caused by poor health, a lack of maternity services, and high levels of infection. Only about 2 percent of Indian women suffer from the kind of infertility that is amenable to ART alone (Qadeer 2009).

3. WHEN THE FISH TALK ABOUT THE WATER

1. UNICEF's Human Rights Council estimates that in India more than 90 percent of people have what is called "arranged marriage," whereby the family, usually the elders, finds the correct match for youngsters of marriageable age (Ghosh 2012).

2. Sterilization is commonly known as "tying tubes" in India due to the practice of tying the fallopian tubes during the procedure. Tubal ligation, or tying of tubes, although medically reversible, requires major surgical intervention, and the reversal operation is not always successful. Women who have undergone tubal ligation or other partial sterilization procedures cannot become traditional surrogates, but can serve as gestational surrogates. Most surrogates in the clinic were not aware that sterilization does not affect the ability to become a gestational surrogate.

4. MANUFACTURING THE PERFECT MOTHER-WORKER

1. There are some exceptions to this unofficial rule. For instance, in the case of two surrogates in this study, the doctor recommended breast-feeding by the surrogate for the sake of the baby's health.
2. It is worth noting that while commercial surrogacy involves an unusual intertwining of women's reproductive capacities with the productive role, there are some fundamental parallels with other forms of work. For example, surrogates, like factory workers, are asked to give up the product of their labor—in one case, a baby, in the other, the surplus value that they produce. In both cases, they are also asked to treat their employer's property as if it were their own, even as they are constantly reminded that it is not.
3. For more on this duality, see Ragone (1994) and Raymond (1990).
4. In chapter 5 I discuss the "gift" narrative in more detail. The language of angelhood is not altogether missing from the surrogacy narratives in India. Instead, idioms like "God's service," "angelhood," and "mission" are evoked by a different set of actors—the brokers and the intended mothers.
5. While Divya insists that nobody at the clinic respects brokers, Vimla states that she has full support of the clinic—the nurses and even Dr. Khanderia. The point here is not about who is correct, but what the narrative shows about the values that Divya is promoting.
6. See, for instance, Honig (1986); Lee Ching (1995); Ngai (2000, 2007).
7. This is partly because these "foreign couples" are ready to spend the extra money for the luxury rooms. The doctor, however, does not offer the luxury rooms to Indian couples even when such a room is unoccupied; instead, the room is reserved for unexpected visits by international clients.

5. EVERYDAY DIVINITIES AND GOD'S LABOR

1. For details of the actual carnage, the role of the state, and the role of the Indian diaspora in the United States, see Kamat and Mathew (2003).
2. Judaism and Islam allow most techniques of assisted reproduction when the egg and sperm originate from the wife and the husband, respectively. In Sunni Islam, third-party donation of any kind (including surrogacy) is not allowed. There is no consensus about the same in Shia Islam, although ethnographic work done by anthropologist Marcia Inhorn indicates that gamete donation happens routinely, albeit secretly in countries like Lebanon. Most scholars indicate that Islam does not permit surrogacy, because of the sacredness of the womb. Attitudes toward reproductive practice vary among Christian groups. While assisted reproduction is not accepted by the Vatican, it may be practiced by Protestant, Anglican, and other denominations. According to traditional Christian views, the embryo has moral status as a human being beginning at conception, and thus most assisted reproductive technologies are forbidden. See Schenker (2005) for a detailed discussion of this point. See also Inhorn (2011).

3. For a fascinating exposition of narratives of creative conception in Hinduism's past, see Bhattacharyya (2006).

4. In this section I have focused on the narratives of transnational clients. None of the Indian clients explicitly used the language of "mission." Some emphasized the "sisterly" relations they had developed with their surrogate and their desire to compensate the surrogate "generously," in both cash and kind.

6. EMBODIED LABOR AND NEO-EUGENICS

1. While corporal feminists (for instance, Elizabeth Grosz [1994] and Iris Marion Young [1990]) tend to have a relatively deeper focus on *embodied* experiences, their emphasis is on embodied experiences within reproduction, pregnancy, and childbirth—the lived, sexed body as experienced from the inside.

2. The phrase "emotional labor" was coined by sociologist Arlie Hochschild in 1983 in her classic book *The Managed Heart*. Work, especially service work, requiring "emotional labor," typically involves face-to-face or voice-to-voice contact, with the aim of inducing particular feelings and responses among those for whom the service is being provided. In *The Managed Heart*, Hochschild looked at how flight attendants engage in emotional labor. In her latest book, *The Outsourced Self: Intimate Life in Market Times* (2012), Hochschild includes dating service providers, wedding planners, professional mourners, and Indian surrogates, to talk about the incursion of the market in many more aspects of "intimate life."

3. For an insightful analysis of older family planning promotional materials and their gendered representations of "Indian modernity," see Chatterjee and Riley (2001).

4. The word *dai* is used interchangeably for a variety of women involved in different aspects of birth-related work. Women in this study used the word to refer to the village midwife as well as the family planning nurse. In some cases, the midwives played the dual role of helping with deliveries and encouraging women to use long-term contraceptives or sterilization (Pinto 2008).

5. In urban areas, a network of government hospitals and urban family welfare centers is primarily responsible for providing family planning methods and services. In rural areas, sterilization and IUD insertions are mostly performed in government hospitals and primary healthcare centers. Occasionally, sterilization camps are organized in rural or urban areas throughout the country.

6. To contextualize the surrogates' decisions to get an abortion, it is worth emphasizing that while the issue of abortion in the global north is linked to women's "right to self-determination" and "the right to choose," in India the liberalization of laws regarding abortion is not linked to feminist activism. The Indian Medical Termination of Pregnancy Act made abortion legal in 1971 and the government often implicitly promotes abortion as a method of family planning (Gupte, Bandewar, and Pisal 1997). The public health services provide abortion for free, but often put pressure on women to adopt a contraceptive method after the abortion.

7. Anthropologist Lawrence Cohen (2005) used the phrase "selective bioavailability" to describe how certain people's bodies are mobilized for the purpose of disaggregation into cells, tissues, and organs, to be used by science and medicine. Cohen used the term in the context of the cross-border organ transplant trade, especially the trade in the organs of people from the global south.

8. Marcia Inhorn (2011) captures a curious instance of this stratification in the market for assisted reproductive technologies in India. She finds that although India is celebrated as a destination for "fertility tourism," some Indian couples are unable to access affordable, high-quality fertility care services in their home country and are thus forced to travel abroad and become what Inhorn calls a class of "reproductive exile."

9. In her book, Twine astutely points out that this stratification is not limited to surrogacy in particular. Most services related to the "reproductive functions of women," whether that is access to contraception or fertility treatments, are very often stratified along these structures.

10. For more on such seemingly contradictory reaction to biomedicalization, see Margaret M. Lock and Patricia Alice Kaufert's edited volume *Pragmatic Women and Body Politics* (2000), which compares the responses of women (in a variety of cultural settings) to modern medical technologies. Several contributors to this volume report similar trends in other countries in the global south.

7. DISPOSABLE WORKERS AND DIRTY LABOR

1. For instance, the catchphrase for the television serial *Mamta* is: "What happens when a woman conspires surrogate pregnancy just out of greed of wealth? What happens when an unhappily married man falls in love with the mother of his surrogate child . . . ?" http://www.bollywoodgate.com/indian-tv-serials/mamta.html. Another serial, *Kkusum*, involves a similar "love" triangle, with the surrogate ultimately marrying the intended father. The surrogate in the popular Bollywood movie *Chori Chori Chupke Chupke* is a prostitute who wreaks havoc by falling in love with the intended father. See also Aditya Bharadwaj (2012), "The Other Mother," for a discussion of the role of popular media in the conflation of prostitutes as providers of "surrogate wombs."

2. Chapter 8 analyzes in more detail the alternative kin networks formed by the surrogates during the period of isolation from their community and family.

8. DISPOSABLE MOTHERS AND KIN LABOR

1. In this landmark custody battle, the surrogate mother, Mary Whitehead, refused to return the baby girl (popularly known as Baby M) to intended parents William and Elizabeth Stern. Baby M was genetically related to both Mary Whitehead and William Stern. According to the contract, Mary was to "relinquish parental rights

and custody of the baby to the Sterns and receive a $10,000 fee for her services." When Mary realized she could not bear to give up the child, she informed the Sterns of her decision and declined the fee. The Sterns went to court in 1987. The New Jersey judge upheld the surrogacy contract and awarded custody of Baby M to the Sterns. "A year later, the New Jersey Supreme Court invalidated the contract, but using the legal standard of best interests of the child, it gave custody to the Sterns" (Markens 2007, 4). Mary Whitehead, however, retained both visitation rights and parental rights.

2. Manji Yamada was born to a gestational surrogate in India in 2007. During the surrogate's pregnancy, the intended parents from Japan got divorced. When Yamada's ex-wife (the intended mother) refused to travel with him to take possession of Manji, he flew to India alone and tried to secure documents to take the baby to Japan. But the Japanese Embassy in India refused to grant Manji a Japanese passport or visa on the grounds that the Japanese Civil Code recognizes only the woman who gives birth to a baby as the mother. The code does not recognize surrogate children. Yamada's next attempt—formally adopting Manji— also did not come to fruition since the Indian Guardians and Wards Act of 1890 does not allow a single man to adopt a baby girl. Yamada ultimately hired one of India's most noted attorneys, who managed to get Manji a birth certificate with only her father's name and a temporary travel document to Japan.

3. For instance, Michael G. Peletz, in a review of kinship studies in the late twentieth century, astutely points out that the emphasis in kinship has shifted to "choice, love and intention" (1995, 365).

4. In her pioneering work, Micaela di Leonardo introduced the concept of "kin work" to refer to the "conception, maintenance, and ritual celebration of cross-household kin ties" (1987, 442). Di Leonardo's concept of kin work made visible an array of tasks culturally assigned to women. Maintaining contacts and a sense of family, di Leonardo argued, takes time, intention, and skill, and should be recognized as work.

5. Wendy Doniger O'Flaherty adds another bodily fluid to this list—the fluid of the womb—lying somewhere between blood and milk. This "mediating fluid" is itself ambiguous and dangerous, and thus establishes only an ambivalent relationship between mother and fetus (1980, 42).

9. CONCLUSION: APORIA OF SURROGACY

1. Pre-implantation genetic diagnosis (PGD) is an embryo screening technique. About three days after fertilization, a single cell is removed from each of the embryos that have been created through in vitro fertilization (IVF). These cells are then tested, and one or more embryos that meet the specified criteria—in the case of sex selection for a boy, those with both X and Y chromosomes—are implanted in a woman's body. The use of PGD adds between $3,000 and $5,000 to the cost of an IVF cycle.

2. A 2012 news report on the surrogacy industry in China confirms this prediction. Although there is no specific law regulating the industry in China, in 2001 the ministry of health banned any trade in fertilized eggs and embryos, which in turn forbids hospitals from performing any gestational surrogacy procedures. The ban is regularly flouted by clinics and clients and has effectively driven the industry underground. While there is no official count of this fledgling industry, a 2011 study estimates that, to date, more than 25,000 children have been born in China through surrogacy arrangements. The article reports that in fact surrogacy is being used by people of higher economic classes to bypass the one-child rule. See http://www.guardian.co.uk/world/2012/feb/08/china-surrogate-mothers-year-dragon.

   A similar controversy was unearthed in Taiwan—where surrogacy is illegal. A surrogacy company based in Taiwan was charged with human trafficking for allegedly holding Vietnamese women in hostels after confiscating their passports. In Guatemala, surrogacy seems to be replacing the industry of international adoptions, which has been featured in the media because of rampant human rights abuses. A *Washington Times* investigation reports that "some of the same people who were arranging international adoptions are acting as surrogacy brokers in Guatemala" (Ehrlich 2011).

3. If one were to read between the lines, the suggested changes sound suspiciously like a misplaced sense of morality. The assumption seems to be that only people in a heterosexual married relationship and people of Indian origin can be trusted to raise children. I have discussed this in greater detail elsewhere (Pande 2013).

4. Humbyrd (2009) outlines in some detail what a formal international agreement governing intercountry surrogacy could look like. She advocates a model similar to the Hague Convention of Intercountry Adoption, as well as more immediate regulations, for instance that clients must work with nationally accredited service providers. Within this regulatory framework, "brokers and agencies involved in international surrogacy could be accredited based on their compliance with Fair Trade surrogacy standards, and the list of approved surrogacy service providers could be publicized on the State Department website as it is for adoption service providers."

5. In her study of domestic work in South Africa, Shireen Ally demonstrates that while the state efforts to modernize and professionalize domestic work as a form of employment in postapartheid South Africa have been remarkable, some domestic workers feel disempowered by these laws. Domestic workers value the intimate negotiations with their employers as much as, if not more than, the rights-based benefits given by the state. When the state positions itself as the representative and protector of the interests of "vulnerable" domestic workers, the workers themselves get demobilized and their voices are muted. Other scholars have reported similar findings. For instance, Latina day workers and part-time cleaners in the studies of Mary Romero (1992) and Leslie Salzinger (1991) are perceived to have "upgraded" the occupation by establishing a businesslike contractual relationship. However, Jennifer Mendez (1998) interviewed cleaners employed by a bureaucratic agency and found that many workers actually prefer private employment, in which they

have the autonomy to select employers and can obtain personal favors. Similarly, Turkish maids and doorkeepers interviewed by Gul Ozyegin (2001) even embrace class hierarchies because they gain raises and extra benefits in a patron-client relationship.

6. See the entire document, which outlines the organization's systematic criticism of the revised ART draft (2010) at http://www.communityhealth.in/~commun26/wiki/images/0/0d/Sama_ART_Bill_Policy_Brief_2010.pdf.

7. Debra Satz (1992) has previously compared surrogacy and adoption and argued for an "open" model: one that regulates the arrangement, that respects the surrogate's option to change her mind, and that provides all relevant details about associated risks.

8. The Hague Convention on Protection of Children and Co-operation in Respect of Inter-country Adoption (1993) seeks to protect children and their families against the risks of illegal, irregular, or ill-prepared adoptions abroad. In India (a signatory to this convention) the Central Adoption Resource Authority (CARA) under the Ministry of Women and Child Development functions as the nodal body for adoption of Indian children. CARA is mandated to monitor and regulate all in-country and inter-country adoptions. See http://adoptionindia.nic.in/guideline-family/Post%20Adoption.html for the specifics on "Root Search," or the rights of the child to obtain information about his or her origins.

9. News reports in 2013 suggest that the regulations passed in 2012 have caused some clients to choose Thailand over India, even though in Thailand the surrogate is listed as the baby's mother on the birth certificate and if she is married, her husband is put down as the father. http://www.abc.net.au/news/2013-04-13/thai-surrogacy-concerns/4624388. Other relevant websites are http://www.ivfmiraclebaby.com/surrogacy.htm for surrogacy in Thailand and http://en.surrogacy-ukraine.com for surrogacy in Ukraine.

10. For instance, in her ethnographic study of residents of shack settlements in post-apartheid South Africa, anthropologist Fiona Ross (2010) reports the importance that the residents place on not just material circumstances but the ability to live in accord with ideals of dignity and decency.

EPILOGUE: DID THE "SPERM ON A RICKSHAW" SAVE THE THIRD WORLD?

1. During the show, the phrase "sperm on a rickshaw" came up as a (jocular) take on men from the United States traveling to clinics in remote parts of India, often in rickshaws, to get tested for infertility.

2. For my visit in 2011, my role as an academic was secondary. I was returning in my capacity as a performer and co-scriptwriter for a multimedia theatrical production from Danish stage director Ditte M. Bjerg and her production house, Global Stories. The ongoing project engages surrogates in hostels in community theater and a livelihood-generating embroidery program. See http://globalstories.net/productions/made-in-india/ and http://madeinindiaglobalstories.wordpress.com/ for more details.

WORKS CITED

Abu-Lughod, Lila. 1990. "The Romance of Resistance: Tracing Transformations of Power Through Bedouin Women." *American Ethnologist* 17 (1): 41–55.

Agrawal, Shraddha, and B. M. Bharti. 2006. "Reproductive Health in Urban Slums." *Journal of Obstetrics and Gynecology of India* 56: 255–57.

Ahluwalia, Sanjam. 2003. "Rethinking Boundaries: Feminism and (Inter)Nationalism in Early-Twentieth-Century India." *Journal of Women's History* 14 (4): 188–95.

Ahmed, Saifuddin, and W. Henry Mosley. 1997. "Simultaneity in Maternal-Child Health Care Utilization and Contraceptive Use: Evidence from Developing Countries." WP97-03, Hopkins Population Center Papers on Population. Baltimore: Department of Population Dynamics, School of Public Health, Johns Hopkins University.

Ali, Lorraine, and Raina Kelley. 2008. "The Curious Lives of Surrogates." *Newsweek*, April 7. Accessed November 28, 2013.

Ali, Syed Intishab. 2011. "Get Sterilized in Rajasthan, Drive Home a Nano." *TNN*, June 30. http://articles.timesofindia.indiatimes.com/2011-06-30/india/29721333_1_nano-car-sterilization-drive-mixer.

Anderson, Elizabeth S. 1990. "Is Women's Labor a Commodity?" *Philosophy and Public Affairs* 19: 71–92.

Anderson, Sandra Vandam, and Eleanor E. Bauwens. 1982. "An Ethnography of Home Birth." In Margarita Artschwager Kay, ed., *Anthropology of Human Birth*. Philadelphia: F. A. Davis.

Andrews, Lori B. 1988. "Surrogate Motherhood: The Challenge for Feminists." *Journal of Law, Medicine, and Ethics* 16 (1–2): 72–80.

Andrews, Lori B., and Lisa Douglass. 1991. "Alternative Reproduction." *Southern California Law Review* 65: 623–82.

Anleu, S. R. 1992. "For Love but Not for Money?" *Gender and Society* 6 (1): 30–48.

Ashforth, Blake E., and Glen E. Kreiner. 1999. " 'How Can You Do It?' Dirty Work and the Challenge of Constructing a Positive Identity." *Academy of Management Review* 24 (3): 413–34.

Bailey, Alison. 2011. "Reconceiving Surrogacy: Toward a Reproductive Justice Account of Indian Surrogacy." In Special FEAST issue, ed. Diane T. Myers. *Hypatia* 26 (4): 715–41.

Baker, Brenda M. 1996. "A Case for Permitting Altruistic Surrogacy." *Hypatia* 11 (2): 34–48.

Bharadwaj, Aditya. 2000. "How Some Indian Baby Makers Are Made: Media Narratives and Assisted Conception in India." *Anthropology and Medicine* 7 (1): 63–78.

——. 2012. "The Other Mother: Supplementary Wombs and the Surrogate State in India." In Michi Knecht, Maren Klotz, and Stefan Beck, eds., *Reproductive Technologies as Global Form: Ethnographies of Knowledge, Practices, and Transnational Encounters*, 139–60. Frankfurt: Campus Verlag.

Bhattacharyya, Swasti. 2006. *Magical Progeny, Modern Technology: A Hindu Bioethics of Assisted Reproductive Technology*. Albany: State University of New York Press.

Black, Paula. 2004. *The Beauty Industry: Gender, Culture, Pleasure*. London: Routledge.

Böck, Monika, and Aparna Rao. 2000. "Indigenous Models and Kinship Theories: An Introduction to a South Asian Perspective." In Monika Böck and Aparna Rao, eds., *Culture, Creation, and Procreation: Concepts of Kinship in South Asian Practice*, 1–49. New York: Berghahn Books.

Bodenhorn, Barbara. 2000. " 'He Used to Be My Relative': Exploring the Bases of Related-ness Among Iñupiat of Northern Alaska." In Janet Carsten, ed., *Cultures of Relatedness: New Approaches to the Study of Kinship*, 128–48. Cambridge, UK: Cambridge University Press.

Boris, Eileen, and Rhacel Salazar Parreñas. 2010. *Intimate Labors: Cultures, Technologies, and the Politics of Care*. Stanford, CA: Stanford University Press

Bornstein, Erica. 2012. *Disquieting Gifts: Humanitarianism in New Delhi*. Stanford, CA: Stanford University Press.

Brennan, Samantha, and Robert Noggle. 1997. "The Moral Status of Children: Children's Rights, Parents' Rights, and Family Justice." *Social Theory and Practice* 23 (1): 1–26.

Briggs, Laura. 2003. "Mother, Child, Race, and Nation: The Visual Iconography of Rescue and the Politics of Transnational and Transracial Adoption." *Gender and History* 15: 179–200.

Brook, Barbara. 1999. *Feminist Perspectives on the Body*. London: Longman.

Burawoy, Michael. 1991. "The Extended Case Method." In Michael Burawoy et al., *Ethnography Unbound: Power and Resistance in the Modern Metropolis*, 271–90. Berkeley: University of California Press

Burkitt, Ian. 1999. *Bodies of Thought: Embodiment, Identity, and Modernity*. London: Sage.

Cannell, Fenella. 1990. "Concepts of Parenthood: The Warnock Report, the Gillick Debate, and Modern Myths." *American Ethnologist* 17: 667–86.

Carney, Scott. 2010. "Inside India's Rent-a-Womb Business." *Mother Jones*, March/April.

Carsten, Janet, ed. 2000. *Cultures of Relatedness: New Approaches to the Study of Kinship*. Cambridge, UK: Cambridge University Press.

Cartwright, Lisa. 2005. "Images of 'Waiting Children': Spectatorship and Pity in the Representation of the Global Social Orphan in the 1990's." In Toby Volkman, ed., *Cultures of Transnational Adoption*, 185–212. Durham, NC: Duke University Press.

Chatterjee, Nilanjana, and Nancy E. Riley. 2001. "Planning an Indian Modernity: The Gendered Politics of Fertility Control." *Signs* 26 (3): 811–45.

Chavkin, Wendy. 2010. Introduction to Wendy Chavkin and JaneMaree Maher, eds., *The Globalization of Motherhood: Deconstructions and Reconstructions of Biology and Care*. New York: Routledge.

Cohen, Lawrence. 2005. "Operability, Bioavailability, and Exception." In Aihwa Ong and Stephen J. Collier, eds., *Global Assemblages: Technology, Politics and Ethics as Anthropological Problems*, 79–90. Malden, MA: Blackwell Publishing.

Cohen, Margot. 2009. "A Search for a Surrogate Leads to India." http://online.wsj.com/article/SB10001424052748704252004574459003279407832.html.

Cole, Jeffrey, and Sally Booth. 2007. *Dirty Work: Immigrants in Domestic Service, Agriculture, and Prostitution in Sicily*. Lanham, MD: Lexington Books.

Colen, Shellee. 1995. "'Like a Mother to Them': Stratified Reproduction and West Indian Childcare Workers and Employers in New York." In Faye Ginsburg and Rayna Rapp, eds., *Conceiving the New World Order: The Global Politics of Reproduction*, 78–102. Berkeley: University of California Press.

Collins, Jane L. 2002. "Mapping a Global Labor Market: Gender and Skill in the Globalizing Garment Industry." *Gender and Society* 16 (6): 921–40.

"Concern Over Draft Health Chapter in Planning Commission Document." 2012. *The Hindu*. Accessed November 28, 2013. http://www.thehindu.com/todays-paper/tp-national/concern-over-draft-health-chapter-in-planning-commission-document/article3752490.ece.

Conly, Shanti R., and Sharon L. Camp. 1992. *India's Family Planning Challenge: From Rhetoric to Action*. Washington, DC: Population Crisis Committee.

Corea, Gena. 1986. *The Mother Machine: Reproductive Technologies from Artificial Insemination to Artificial Wombs*. New York: HarperCollins.

Daniel, E. Valentine. 1984. *Fluid Signs: Being a Person the Tamil Way*. Berkeley: University of California Press.

Das, Abhijit. 2003. "Two Children, Countless Wrongs." *India Together*. www.indiatogether.org/2003./oct/hlt-twokids.htm. October.

Das, N. P., Vinod K. Mishra, and P. K. Saha. 2001. "Does Community Access Affect the Use of Health and Family Welfare Services in Rural India?" National Family Health Survey Subject Reports No. 18. Mumbai: International Institute for Population Sciences; and Honolulu: East-West Center.

DasGupta, Sayantani, and Shamita Das Dasgupta. 2010. "Motherhood Jeopardized: Reproductive Technologies in Indian Communities." In Wendy Chavkin and JaneMaree Maher, eds., *The Globalization of Motherhood: Deconstructions and Reconstructions of Biology and Care*, 131–53. New York: Routledge.

——, eds. 2014. *Globalization and Gestational Surrogacy in India: Outsourcing Life*. New York: Lexington Books.

Davis-Floyd, Robbie. 1990. "The Role of American Obstetrics in the Resolution of Cultural Anomaly." *Social Science and Medicine* 31:175–189.

Dharmalingam, A. 1995. "The Social Context of Family Planning in a South Indian Village." *International Family Planning Perspectives* 1 (3): 98–103.

di Leonardo, Micaela. 1987. "The Female World of Cards and Holidays: Women, Families, and the Work of Kinship." *Signs* 12 (3): 440–53.

Douglas, Mary. 2002. *Purity and Danger: An Analysis of the Concepts of Pollution and Taboo.* London: Routledge Classics.

Dube, Leela. 1986. "Seed and Earth: The Symbolism of Biological Reproduction and Sexual Relations of Production." In Leela Dube, Eleanor Leacock, and Shirley Ardener, eds., *Visibility and Power: Essays on Women in Society and Development*, 22–41. Delhi: Oxford University Press.

——. 2001. *Anthropological Explorations in Gender: Intersecting Fields.* New Delhi: Sage.

Dublin, Thomas. 1975. "Women, Work, and the Family: Female Operatives in the Lowell Mills, 1830–1860." *Feminist Studies* 3 (1/2): 30–39.

Dworkin, Andrea. 1978. *Right-Wing Women.* New York: Perigee Books.

Ehrlich, Richard S. 2011. "Thai Company Accused of Trafficking Vietnamese Women to Breed." *Washington Times*, March 7.

Ekman, Kajsa Ekis. 2011. *Varat och varan: Prostitution, surrogatmödraskap och den delade människan.* Stockholm: Leopard.

Franklin, Sarah, and Celia Roberts. 2006. *Born and Made: An Ethnography of Preimplantation Genetic Diagnosis.* Princeton, NJ: Princeton University Press.

Fraser, Nancy. 2011. "Between Marketisation and Social Protection: Ambivalences of Feminism in the Context of Capitalist Crisis." Humanitas Lecture 3, University of Cambridge. Accessed September 15, 2011. www.crassh.cam.ac.uk/events/1536.

Freeman, Carla. 2000. *High Tech and High Heels in the Global Economy.* Durham, NC: Duke University Press.

Fruzzetti, Lina, and Ákos Östör. 1984. *Kinship and Ritual in Bengal: Anthropological Essays.* New Delhi: South Asian Publisher Pvt., Ltd.

Gamburd, Michele Ruth. 2000. *The Kitchen Spoon's Handle.* Ithaca, NY: Cornell University Press.

George, Sheba. 2000. "'Dirty Nurses' and 'Men Who Play.'" In Burawoy et al., *Global Ethnography: Forces, Connections, and Imaginations in a Postmodern World*, 144–74. Berkeley: University of California Press.

Ghosh, Palash. 2012. "Indian Village Bans 'Love Marriages,' But Arranged Marriages Remains the Norm Anyway." http://www.ibtimes.com/indian-village-bans-love-marriages-arranged-marriages-remains-norm-anyway-723314.

Gibbon, Sahra, and Carlos Novas. 2008. Introduction to *Biosocialities, Genetics, and the Social Sciences—Making Biologies and Identities.* London: Routledge.

Gimlin, Debra L. 2002. *Body Work: Beauty and Self-Image in American Culture.* Berkeley: University of California Press.

Ginsburg, Faye, and Rayna Rapp. 1991. "The Politics of Reproduction." *Annual Review of Anthropology* 20: 311–43.

Glenn, Evelyn Nakano. 1992. "From Servitude to Service Work: Historical Continuities in the Racial Division of Paid Reproduction Labor." *Signs* 18: 1–43.

Goffman, Erving. 1963. *Stigma: Notes on the Management of Spoiled Identity.* Englewood Cliffs, NJ: Prentice-Hall.

Govindasamy, Pavalavalli. 2000. "Poverty, Women's Education, and Utilization of Health Services in Egypt." In Brígida Garcia, ed., *Women, Poverty, and Demographic Change*, 263–85. New York: Oxford University Press.

Govindasamy, Pavalavalli, and B. M. Ramesh. 1997. *Maternal Education and the Utilization of Maternal and Child Health Services in India.* National Family Health Survey Subject Reports, no. 5. Mumbai: International Institute for Population Sciences; and Calverton: Macro International, Demographic and Health Surveys (DHS).

Grosz, Elizabeth. 1994. *Volatile Bodies. Toward a Corporeal Feminism.* Bloomington: Indiana University Press.

Gruenbaum, Ellen. 1998. "Resistance and Embrace: Sudanese Rural Women and Systems of Power." In Margaret Lock and Patricia Kaufert, eds., *Pragmatic Women and Body Politics,* 58–76. Cambridge, UK: Cambridge University Press.

Gupta, Jyotsna Agnihotri. 2006. "Towards Transnational Feminisms: Some Reflections and Concerns in Relation to the Globalization of Reproductive Technologies." *European Journal of Women's Studies* 13 (1): 23–38.

——. 2012. "Reproductive Biocrossings: Indian Egg Donors and Surrogates in the Globalized Fertility Market." *International Journal of Feminist Approaches to Bioethics* 5 (1): 25–51.

Gupte, Manisha, Sunita Bandewar, and Hemlata Pisal. 1997. "Abortion Needs of Women in India: A Case Study of Rural Maharashtra." *Reproductive Health Matters* 5 (9): 77–86.

Haimowitz, Rebecca, and Vaishali Sinha. 2010. *Made in India.* Dir: Vaishali Sinha|Rebecca Haimowitz/Hindi|English/97min/2010.

Harding, Sandra. 1991. *Whose Science? Whose Knowledge? Thinking from Women's Lives.* Ithaca, NY: Cornell University Press.

Hartmann, Betsy. 1995. *Reproductive Rights and Wrongs: The Global Politics of Population Control.* Cambridge, MA: South End Press.

——. 2006. "Eugenics of the Everyday: Some Preliminary Reflections." Background paper for the Consultation on New Reproductive and Genetic Technologies and Women's Lives, New Delhi, June.

——. 2010. "The Gene Express: Speeding Towards What Future?" In *Unravelling the Fertility Industry: Challenges and Strategies for Movement Building.* A report based on an International Consultation on Commercial, Economic, and Ethical Aspects of Assisted Reproductive Technologies. Delhi: SAMA Resource Group for Women and Health.

Hazarika, Indrajit. 2010. "Women's Reproductive Health in Slum Populations in India: Evidence from NFHS-3." *Journal of Urban Health* 87 (2): 264–77.

Heng, B. C. 2007. "Regulatory Safeguards Needed for the Traveling Foreign Egg Donor." *Human Reproduction* 22 (8): 2350–52.

Hershman, Paul. 1981. *Punjabi Kinship and Marriage.* Delhi: Hindustan Publishing.

Hochschild, Arlie Russell. 1983. *The Managed Heart: Commercialization of Human Feeling.* Berkeley: University of California Press.

——. 2009. "Childbirth at the Global Crossroads." *American Prospect,* October 5.

——. 2012. *The Outsourced Self: Intimate Life in Market Times.* New York: Metropolitan Books.

Hollander, Jocelyn A., and Rachel L. Einwohner. 2004. "Conceptualizing Resistance." *Sociological Forum* 19 (4): 533–554.

Hondagneu-Sotelo, Pierrette, and Ernestine Avila. 1997. " 'I'm Here, but I'm There': The Meaning of Latina Transnational Motherhood." *Gender and Society* 11 (5): 548–71.

Honig, Emily. 1986. *Sisters and Strangers: Women in the Shanghai Cotton Mills, 1919–1949.* Stanford, CA: Stanford University Press.

Humbyrd, Casey. 2009. "Fair Trade International Surrogacy." *Developing World Bioethics* 9 (3): 111–18.

Inden, Ronald B., and Ralph W. Nicholas. 1977. *Kinship in Bengali Culture*. Chicago: University of Chicago Press.

Inhorn, Marcia. 2010. "Assisted Motherhood in Global Dubai: Reproductive Tourists and Their Helpers." In Wendy Chavkin and JaneMaree Maher, eds., *The Globalization of Motherhood: Deconstructions and Reconstructions of Biology and Care*, 180–202. New York: Routledge.

——. 2011. "Globalization and Gametes: Reproductive 'Tourism,' Islamic Bioethics, and Middle Eastern Modernity." *Anthropology and Medicine* 18 (1): 87–103.

Jaggar, Alison M., and Susan R. Bordo, eds. 1989. *Gender/Body/Knowledge: Feminist Reconstructions of Being and Knowing*. New Brunswick, NJ: Rutgers University Press.

"Japanese Baby Gets Birth Certificate." 2008. *The Hindu*, August 11. Accessed November 13, 2010. http://www.thehindu.com/2008/08/11/stories/2008081160180300.htm.

Jeffery, Patricia. 2001. "Agency, Activism, and Agendas." In Patricia Jeffery and Amrita Basu, eds., *Resisting the Sacred and the Secular: Women's Activism and Political Religion*, 221–43. New Delhi: Kali for Women.

Jeffery, Patricia, Roger Jeffery, and A. Lyon. 1989. *Labour Pains, Labour Power: Women and Childbearing in India*. London: Zed Books.

Jolly, Margaret, and Kalpana Ram, eds. 2001. *Borders of Being: Citizenship, Fertility, and Sexuality in Asia and the Pacific*. Ann Arbor: University of Michigan Press.

Kamat, Sangeeta, and Biju Mathew. 2003. "Mapping Political Violence in a Globalized World: The Case of Hindu Nationalism." *Social Justice* 30: 4–16.

Kang, Miliann. 2003. "The Managed Hand: The Commercialization of Bodies and Emotions in Korean Immigrant-Owned Nail Salons." *Gender and Society* 17 (6): 820–39.

Kanitkar, Tara, and R. K. Sinha. 1989. "Antenatal Care Services in Five States of India." In S. N. Singh, M. K. Premi, P. S. Bhatia, and Ashish Bose, eds., *Population Transition in India*, 2: 201–11. Delhi: B. R. Publishing.

Kannan, Shilpa. 2009. "Regulators Eye India's Surrogacy Sector." *India Business Report, BBC World*, March 18. Accessed April 8, 2009. http://news.bbc.co.uk/2/hi/business/7935768.htm.

Karkal, Malini. 1998. "Family Planning and the Reproductive Rights of Women." In Lakshmi Lingam, ed., *Understanding Women's Health Issues: A Reader*, 228. New Delhi: Kali.

Khare, R. S. 1992. "From Kanya to Mata: Aspects of the Cultural Language of Kinship in Northern India." In Akos Ostor, Lina Fruzzetti, and Steve Barnett, eds., *Concepts of Person: Kinship, Caste, and Marriage in India*, 143–71. Cambridge, MA: Harvard University Press.

Kohli, Namita. 2011. "Moms on the Market." *Hindustan Times*, March.

Krishnakumar, Asha. 2003. "The Science of ART." *Frontline* 20:19.

Krishnan, Prabha. 1990. "In the Idiom of Loss: Ideology of Motherhood in Television Serials." *Economic and Political Weekly* 25 (42–43): 103–15.

Kumar, Anand T. C. 2007. "Ethical Aspects of Assisted Reproduction: An Indian Viewpoint." *Reproductive BioMedicine Online* 14 (1): 140–42.

Kumar, Pushpesh. 2006. "Gender and Procreative Ideologies Among the Kolams of Maharashtra." *Contributions to Indian Sociology* 40: 279.

Lambert, Helen. 1996. "Caste, Gender, and Locality in Rural Rajasthan." In C. J. Fuller, ed., *Caste Today*, 93–123. Delhi: Oxford University Press.

——. 2000. "Village Bodies? Reflection on Locality, Constitution, and Affect in Rajasthani Kinship." In Monica Böck and Aparna Rao, eds., *Culture, Creation, and Procreation: Concepts of Kinship in South Asian Practice*, 81–100. New York: Berghahn Books.

Lamont, Michèle. 2000. *The Dignity of Working Men: Morality and the Boundaries of Race, Class, and Immigration.* New York: Russell Sage Foundation.

Lamont, Michèle, and Marcel Fournier, eds. 1992. *Cultivating Differences: Symbolic Boundaries and the Making of Inequality.* Chicago: University of Chicago Press.

Layne, Linda. 1999. *Transformative Motherhood: On Giving and Getting in a Consumer Culture.* New York: NYU Press.

Lee Ching, Kwan. 1995. "Engendering the Worlds of Labor: Women Workers, Labor Markets, and Production Politics in the South China Economic Miracle." *American Sociological Review* 60: 378–97.

Levine, Hal B. 2003. "Gestational Surrogacy: Nature and Culture in Kinship." *Ethnology* 42: 173–85.

Lock, Margaret, and Patricia A. Kaufert, eds. 2000. *Pragmatic Women and Body Politics.* Cambridge, UK: Cambridge University Press.

Madan, T. N. 1981. "The Ideology of the Householder Among the Kashmiri Pandits." *Contributions to Indian Sociology* 15 (1–2): 223–50.

Malpani, A., A. Malpani, and D. Modi. 2002. "Preimplantation Sex Selection for Family Balancing in India." *Human Reproduction* 17 (1): 11–12.

Markens, Susan. 2007. *Surrogate Motherhood and the Politics of Reproduction.* Berkeley: University of California Press.

Martin, Emily. 2001. *The Woman in the Body: A Cultural Analysis of Reproduction.* Boston: Beacon Press.

Mavalankar, Dileep, and Kranti Suresh Vora. 2008. "The Changing Role of Auxiliary Nurse Midwife (ANM) in India: Implications for Maternal and Child Health." Working Paper No. 2008-03-01, Indian Institute of Management Ahmedabad, Ahmedabad, Gujarat, India.

McCormack, Karen. 2005. "Stratified Reproduction and Poor Women's Resistance." *Gender and Society* 19 (5): 660–79.

Meillassoux, Claude. 1981. *Maidens, Meal, and Money: Capitalism and the Domestic Community.* Cambridge, UK: Cambridge University Press.

Mendez, Jennifer Bickham. 1998. "Of Mops and Maids: Contradictions and Continuities in Bureaucratized Domestic Work." *Social Problems* 45: 114–35.

Mies, Maria. 1986. *Patriarchy and Accumulation on a World Scale: Women in the International Division of Labour.* London: Zed Books.

Mies, Maria, and Vandana Shiva. 1993. *Ecofeminism.* Melbourne: Spinifex.

Mishra, Vinod, and Robert D. Retherford. 2008. "The Effect of Antenatal Care on Professional Assistance at Delivery in Rural India." *Population Research and Policy Review* 27 (3): 307–20.

Mistry, Ritesh, Osman Galal, and Michael Lu. 2009. "Women's Autonomy and Pregnancy Care in Rural India: A Contextual Analysis." *Social Science and Medicine* 69 (6): 926–33.

Mohanty, Chandra Talpade. 2003. *Feminism Without Borders: Decolonizing Theory, Practicing Solidarity.* Durham, NC: Duke University Press.

Mony, P. K., L. Verghese, S. Bhattacharji, A. George, P. Thoppuram, and M. Mathai. 2006. "Demography, Environmental Status, and Maternal Health Care in Slums of Vellore Town, Southern India." *Indian Journal of Community Medicine* 31: 230–33.

Mumby, Dennis K. 2005. "Theorizing Resistance in Organization Studies: A Dialectical Approach." *Management Communication Quarterly* 19: 1–26.

Munjial, Monica, Poonam Kaushik, and Sunil Agnihotri. 2009. "A Comparative Analysis of Institutional and Non-institutional Deliveries in a Village of Punjab Health and Population." *Perspectives and Issues* 32 (3): 131–40.

Narayana, G., and John F. Kantner. 1992. *Doing the Needful: The Dilemma of India's Population Policy.* Boulder, CO: Westview.

Navaneetham, K., and A. Dharmalingam. 2002. "Utilization of Maternal Health Care Services in Southern India." *Social Science and Medicine* 55 (10): 1849–69.

Neuhaus, Richard John. 1988. "Renting Women, Buying Babies, and Class Struggles." *Society* 25 (3): 8–10.

Ngai, Pun. 2000. *Made in China: Women Factory Workers in the Global Workplace.* Chicago: University of Chicago Press.

——. 2007. "Gendering the Dormitory Labor System: Production, Reproduction, and Migrant Labor in South China." *Feminist Economics* 13 (3): 239–58.

Oerton, Sarah, and Joanna Phoenix. 2001. "Sex/Bodywork: Discourses and Practices." *Sexualities* 4 (4): 387–412.

O'Flaherty, Wendy Doniger. 1980. *Women, Androgynes, and Other Mythical Beasts.* Chicago: University of Chicago Press.

Oliver, Kelly. 1989. "Marxism and Surrogacy." *Hypatia* 4 (3): 95–115.

Ong, Aihwa. 1987. *Spirit of Resistance and Capitalist Discipline: Factory Women in Malaysia.* Albany: State University of New York Press.

Ozyegin, Gul. 2001. *Untidy Gender: Domestic Work in Turkey.* Philadelphia: Temple University Press.

Pande, Amrita. 2009a. " 'It May Be Her Eggs but It's My Blood': Surrogates and Everyday Forms of Kinship in India." *Qualitative Sociology* 32 (4): 379–405.

——. 2009b. "Not an 'Angel,' Not a 'Whore': Surrogates as 'Dirty' Workers in India." *Indian Journal of Gender Studies* 16 (2): 141–73.

——. 2010a. "At Least I Am Not Sleeping with Anyone." In "Special Issue on Reproduction and Mothering," *Feminist Studies* 36 (2): 292–312,

——. 2010b. "Commercial Surrogacy in India: Manufacturing a Perfect 'Mother-Worker.' " *Signs: Journal of Women in Culture and Society* 35 (4): 969–94.

——. 2011. "Transnational Commercial Surrogacy in India: Gifts for Global Sisters?" in special issue, *Reproductive BioMedicine Online* 23 (5): 618–25.

——. 2013. "An Infantile Idea?" August 13, 2013. http://www.indianexpress.com/news/an-infantile-idea/1155935/.

Parreñas, Rhacel Salazar. 2005. *Children of Global Migration: Transnational Families and Gendered Woes.* Stanford, CA: Stanford University Press.

Pateman, Carole. 1988. *The Sexual Contract.* Stanford, CA: Stanford University Press, 1988.

Peletz, Michael G. 1995. "Kinship Studies in Late Twentieth-Century Anthropology." *Annual Review of Anthropology* 24: 343–72.

Pennings, Guido. 2002. "Reproductive Tourism as Moral Tourism in Motion." *Journal of Medical Ethics* 28: 337–41.

Petchesky, Rosalind Pollack. 1995. "The Body as a Property: A Feminist Re-vision." In Faye Ginsburg and Rayna Rapp, eds., *Conceiving the New World Order: The Global Politics of Reproduction*, 387–406. Berkeley: University of California Press.

Pinto, Sarah. 2008. *Where There Is No Midwife: Birth and Loss in Rural India.* New York: Berghahn Books.

Planning Commission of India. 2012. "Press Note on Poverty Estimates, 2009–10." http://planningcommission.nic.in/news/press_pov1903.pdf.

Qadeer, Imrana. 2009. "Social and Ethical Basis of Legislation on Surrogacy: Need for Debate." *Indian Journal of Medical Ethics* 6 (1): 2832. Mumbai: Forum for Medical Ethics Society.

——. 2010a. "The ART of Marketing Babies." *Indian Journal of Medical Ethics* 7 (4): 209–15.

——. 2010b. *New Reproductive Technologies and Health Care in Neo-liberal India: Essays.* New Delhi: Centre for Women's Development Studies.

Rabinow, Paul. 1996. "Artificiality and Enlightenment: From Sociobiology to Biosociality." In *Essays on the Anthropology of Reason*, 91–112. Princeton, NJ: Princeton University Press.

Radin, Margaret Jane. 1987. "Market–Inalienability." *Harvard Law Review* 100 (8): 1849–1937.

Ragoné, Helena. 1994. *Surrogate Motherhood: Conception in the Heart.* Boulder, CO: Westview.

Raheja, Gloria Goodwin, and Ann Grodzins Gold. 1994. *Listen to the Heron's Words: Reimagining Gender and Kinship in North India.* Berkeley: University of California Press.

Rajadhyaksha, Madhavi. 2013. "No Surrogacy Visa for Gay Foreigners." Accessed November 28, 2013. http://articles.timesofindia.indiatimes.com/2013-01-18/india/36415052_1_surrogacy-fertility-clinics-home-ministry.

Ram, Kalpana. 2001. "Rationalizing Fecund Bodies: Family Planning Policy and the Modern Indian Nation-State." In Margaret Jolly and Kalpana Ram, eds., *Borders of Being: Citizenship, Fertility, and Sexuality in Asia and the Pacific*, 82–117. Ann Arbor: University of Michigan Press.

Ramesh, Randeep. 2006. "British Couples Desperate for Children Travel to India in Search of Surrogates." *Guardian*, March 20.

Rao, Mohan, ed. 2004. *The Unheard Scream: Reproductive Health and Women's Lives in India.* New Delhi: Zubaan.

Rapp, Rayna. 2001. "Gender, Body, Biomedicine: How Some Feminist Concerns Dragged Reproduction to the Center of Social Theory." *Medical Anthropology Quarterly* 15 (4): 466–77.

Raymond, Janice G. 1990. "Reproductive Gifts and Gift Giving: The Altruistic Woman." *Hastings Center Report* 20 (6): 7–11.

——. 1993. *Women as Wombs: Reproductive Technologies and the Battle Over Women's Freedom.* San Francisco: HarperSanFrancisco; Melbourne: Spinifex Press; Munich: Frauenoffensive.

Remez, L. 2001. "Prevention of Unwanted Births in India Would Result in Replacement Fertility." *International Family Planning Perspectives* 27 (2): 104.

Roberts, Dorothy. 1997. *Killing the Black Body: Race, Reproduction, and the Meaning of Liberty.* New York: Pantheon.

——. 2009. "Race, Gender, and Genetic Technologies: A New Reproductive Dystopia?" *Signs* 34 (4): 783–804.

Robertson, John A. 2004. "Protecting Embryos and Burdening Women: Assisted Reproduction in Italy." *Human Reproduction* 19 (4): 1693–96.

Romero, Mary. 1992. *Maid in the U.S.A.* London and New York: Routledge.

Ross, Fiona. 2010. *Raw Life, New Hope: Decency, Housing, and Everyday Life in a Post-apartheid Community.* Cape Town: UCT Press

Rotabi, Karen Smith, and Nicole Footen Bromfield. 2012. "The Decline in Intercountry Adoptions and New Practices of Global Surrogacy: Global Exploitation and Human Rights Concerns." *Affilia* 27: 129–41.

Rothman, Barbara Katz. 1982. *In Labor: Women and Power in the Birthplace.* New York: W. W. Norton.

——. 1986. *The Tentative Pregnancy: How Amniocentesis Changes the Experience of Motherhood.* New York: Viking.

——. 1988. "Reproductive Technology and the Commodification of Life." In Elaine Hoffman Baruch, Amadeo F. D'Adamo Jr., and Joni Seager, eds., *Embryos, Ethics, and Women's Rights: Exploring the New Reproductive Technologies*, 95–100, New York: Hawthorn Press.

——. 1989. "Women as Fathers: Motherhood and Child Care Under a Modified Patriarchy." *Gender and Society* 3 (1): 89–104.

——. 2000. *Recreating Motherhood: Ideology and Technology in a Patriarchal Society.* New Brunswick, NJ: Rutgers University Press. First published 1989 by W. W. Norton.

Rudrappa, Sharmila. 2012. "India's Reproductive Assembly Line." *Contexts* 11 (2): 22–27.

Rutenberg, Naomi, and Evelyn Landry. 1993. "A Comparison of Sterilization Use and Demand from the Demographic and Health Surveys." *International Family Planning Perspectives* 19 (1): 4–13.

Salzinger, Leslie. 1991. "A Maid by Any Other Name: The Transformation of 'Dirty Work' by Central American Immigrants." In Michael Burawoy et al., *Ethnography Unbound: Power and Resistance in Modern Metropolis*, 139–60. Berkeley: University of California Press.

——. 1993. *Genders in Production: Making Workers in Mexico's Global Factories.* Berkeley: University of California Press.

SAMA—Resource Group for Women and Health. 2010. The Assisted Reproductive Technologies (Regulation) Bill and Rules (Draft) –2010 Issues and Concerns. http://www.communityhealth.in/~commun26/wiki/images/0/0d/Sama_ART_Bill_Policy_Brief_2010.pdf.

SAMA Women's Health Group. 2010. *Unravelling the Fertility Industry: Challenges and Strategies for Movement Building.* Report of International Consultation. Delhi: Author.

——. 2012. *Birthing a Market: A Study on Commercial Surrogacy*. New Delhi: Author.

Saravanan, Sheela. 2010. "Transnational Surrogacy and Objectification of Gestational Mothers." *Economic and Political Weekly* 45 (16): 26–29.

Saroha, Ekta, Maja Altarac, and Lynn M. Sibley. 2008. "Caste and Maternal Health Care Service Use Among Rural Hindu Women in Maitha, Uttar Pradesh, India." *Journal of Midwifery and Women's Health* 53 (5): 41–47.

Satz, D. 1992. "Markets in Women's Reproductive Labor." *Philosophy and Public Affairs* 21 (2): 107–31.

——. 2010. *Why Some Things Should Not Be for Sale: The Moral Limits of Markets*. New York: Oxford University Press.

Sax, William. 1991. *Mountain Goddess: Gender and Politics in a Himalayan Pilgrimage*. New York: Oxford University Press.

Schenker, Joseph G. 2005. "Assisted Reproduction Practice: Religious Perspectives." *Reproductive BioMedicine Online* 10 (3): 310–19.

Scheper-Hughes, Nancy. 1992 *Death Without Weeping: The Violence of Everyday Life in Brazil*. Berkeley: University of California Press.

Schneider, David M. 1984. *A Critique of the Study of Kinship*. Ann Arbor: University of Michigan Press.

Scott, James C. 1985. *Weapons of the Weak: Everyday Forms of Peasant Resistance*. New Haven, CT: Yale University Press.

Sengupta, Amit. 2010. "Technology, Markets, and the Commoditisation of Life." In *Unravelling the Fertility Industry: Challenges and Strategies for Movement Building*. A report based on an International Consultation on Commercial, Economic, and Ethical Aspects of Assisted Reproductive Technologies. Delhi: SAMA Resource Group for Women and Health.

Shariff, Abusaleh. 1993. "Determinants of Child Health: Search for Maternal Education Effects in Gujarat." Working Paper No. 47, Ahmedabad: Gujarat Institute of Development Research.

Shariff, Abusaleh, and Geeta Singh. 2002. "Determinants of Maternal Health Care Utilisation in India: Evidence from a Recent Household Survey." Working Paper Series No. 85, National Council of Applied Economic Research, New Delhi.

Sharp, Lesley. 2000. "The Commodification of the Body and Its Parts." *Annual Review of Anthropology* 29: 287–328.

Shilling, Chris. 1993. *The Body and Social Theory*. London: Sage.

Spar, Debora L. 2006. *The Baby Business: How Money, Science, and Politics Drive the Commerce of Conception*. Cambridge, MA: Harvard Business Review Press.

Stern, Alexandra Minna. 2005. *Eugenic Nation: Faults and Frontiers of Better Breeding in Modern America*. Berkeley: University of California Press.

Storrow, Richard F. 2010. "The Pluralism Problem in Cross-Border Reproductive Care." *Human Reproduction* 25 (12): 2939–43.

Strathern, Marilyn. 1988. *The Gender of the Gift: Problems with Women and Problems with Society in Melanesia*. Berkeley: University of California Press.

——. 1992. *Reproducing the Future: Essays on Anthropology, Kinship, and the New Reproductive Technologies*. Manchester: Manchester University Press.

"Surrogate Mother Dies of Complications." 2012. *Times News Network.* Accessed November 28, 2013. http://articles.timesofindia.indiatimes.com/2012–05–17/ahmedabad/31748277_1_surrogate-mother-surrogacy-couples.

Sutherland, Gail Hinich. 1990. "*Bīja* (Seed) and *Kṣ Etra* (Field): Male Surrogacy or *Niyoga* in the Mahābhārata'. *Contributions to Indian Sociology* 24 (1): 77–103.

Sykes, Gresham M., and David Matza. 1957. "Techniques of Neutralization: A Theory of Delinquency." *American Sociological Review* 22: 664–70.

Teman, Elly. 2006. "The Birth of a Mother: Mythologies of Surrogate Motherhood in Israel." Ph.D. diss., Hebrew University of Jerusalem.

——. 2010. *Birthing a Mother: The Surrogate Body and the Pregnant Self.* Berkeley: University of California Press.

Thapan, Meenakshi. 2009. *Living the Body: Embodiment, Womanhood, and Identity in Contemporary India.* New Delhi: Sage.

Thompson, Charis. 2005. *Making Parents: The Ontological Choreography of Reproductive Technologies.* Cambridge, MA: MIT Press.

Thompson, E. P. 1978. "Eighteenth-Century English Society: Class Struggle Without Class." *Social History* 3 (2): 133–65.

Trautmann, Thomas. 1981. *Dravidian Kinship.* Cambridge, UK: Cambridge University Press.

Turner, Bryan S. 1984. *The Body and Society: Explorations in Social Theory.* Oxford: Blackwell.

Twigg, Julia. 2000. "Care Work as a Form of Body Work." *Ageing and Society* 20: 389–411.

Twine, France Winddance. 2011. *Outsourcing the Womb: Race, Class, and Gestational Surrogacy in a Global Market.* Framing 21st Century Social Issues. New York: Routledge.

Unnithan, Maya. 2010. "Infertility and Assisted Reproductive Technologies (ARTs) in a Globalising India: Ethics, Medicalization, and Agency." *Asian Bioethics Review* 2 (1): 3–18.

"U.S. Woman Advised to Bring Husband or Adopt Surrogate Baby." 2012. *The Hindu,* January 29. http://www.the.com/news/cities/Hyderabad/article2842743.ece.

Van Hollen, Cecilia.1998 "Moving Targets: Routine IUD Insertion in Maternity Wards in Tamil Nadu, India." *Reproductive Health Matters* 6 (11): 98–106.

——. 2003. "Invoking Vali: Painful Technologies of Modern Birth in South India." *Medical Anthropology Quarterly* 17 (l): 49–77.

Vatuk, Sylvia. 1975. "Gifts and Affines in North India." *Contributions to Indian Sociology* 9: 155–96.

Visaria, Leela, Akash Acharya, and Francis Raj. 2006. "Two-Child Norm Victimising the Vulnerable?" *Economic and Political Weekly,* January 7.

Visaria, Pravin. 2002. "Population Policy." *Seminar,* no. 511.

Volkman, Toby Alice. 2005. "Introduction: New Geographies of Kinship." In Toby Alice Volkman, ed., *Cultures of Transnational Adoption,* 1–24. Durham, NC: Duke University Press.

Vora, Kalindi. 2010. "Medicine, Markets, and the Pregnant Body: Indian Commercial Surrogacy and Reproductive Labor in a Transnational Frame." *Scholar and Feminist Online.*

——. 2012. "Limits of Labor: Accounting for Affect and the Biological in Transnational Surrogacy and Service Work." *South Atlantic Quarterly* 111 (4): 681–700.

Warnock, Mary. 1985. *A Question of Life: The Warnock Report on Fertilization and Embryology.* Cambridge, UK: Blackwell Publishers.

Weitz, Rose, ed. 2003. *The Politics of Women's Bodies: Sexuality, Appearance, and Behaviour.* New York: Oxford University Press.

Whittaker, Andrea, and Amy Speier. 2010. "Cycling Overseas: Care, Commodification, and Stratification in Cross-Border Reproductive Travel." *Medical Anthropology* 29 (4): 363–83.

Witz, Anne M., Chris Warhurst, and Dennis P. Nickson. 2003. "The Labour of Aesthetics and the Aesthetics of Organisation." *Organisation* 10 (1): 33–54.

Wolkowitz, Carol. 2006. *Bodies at Work.* London: Sage.

Wright, Melissa W. 2006. *Disposable Women and Other Myths of Global Capitalism.* New York: Routledge.

Young, Iris Marion. 1990. *Throwing Like a Girl and Other Essays in Feminist Philosophy and Social Theory.* Bloomington: Indiana University Press.

Zavier, Francis, and Sabu S. Padmadas. 2000. "Use of a Spacing Method Before Sterilization Among Couples in Kerala, India." *International Family Planning Perspectives* 26 (1): 29–35.

Zelizer, Viviana A. 1985. *Pricing the Priceless Child: The Changing Social Value of Children.* Princeton, NJ: Princeton University Press.

INDEX

SOUTH ASIA ACROSS THE DISCIPLINES